Coagulopathy

Editors

JEFFREY D. BENNETT
ELIE M. FERNEINI

ORAL AND MAXILLOFACIAL SURGERY CLINICS OF NORTH AMERICA

www.oralmaxsurgery.theclinics.com

Consulting Editor
RICHARD H. HAUG

November 2016 • Volume 28 • Number 4

ELSEVIER

1600 John F. Kennedy Boulevard • Suite 1800 • Philadelphia, Pennsylvania, 19103-2899

http://www.oralmaxsurgery.theclinics.com

ORAL AND MAXILLOFACIAL SURGERY CLINICS OF NORTH AMERICA Volume 28, Number 4
November 2016 ISSN 1042-3699, ISBN-13: 978-0-323-47691-1

Editor: John Vassallo; j.vassallo@elsevier.com
Developmental Editor: Colleen Viola

Oral and Maxillofacial Surgery Clinics of North America (ISSN 1042-3699) is published quarterly by Elsevier Inc., 360 Park Avenue South, New York, NY 10010-1710. Months of issue are February, May, August, and November. Business and Editorial Offices: 1600 John F. Kennedy Blvd., Suite 1800, Philadelphia, PA 19103-2899. Periodicals postage paid at New York, NY and additional mailing offices. Subscription prices are $385.00 per year for US individuals, $628.00 per year for US institutions, $100.00 per year for US students and residents, $455.00 per year for Canadian individuals, $753.00 per year for Canadian institutions, $520.00 per year for international individuals, $753.00 per year for international institutions and $235.00 per year for Canadian and foreign students/residents. To receive student/resident rate, orders must be accompanied by name or affiliated institution, date of term, and the *signature* of program/residency coordinator on institution letterhead. Orders will be billed at individual rate until proof of status is received. Foreign air speed delivery is included in all *Clinics* subscription prices. All prices are subject to change without notice. **POSTMASTER:** Send address changes to *Oral and Maxillofacial Surgery Clinics of North America,* Elsevier Periodicals **Customer Service, 11830 Westline Industrial Drive, St. Louis, MO 63146. Tel: 1-800-654-2452 (U.S. and Canada); 314-447-8871 (outside U.S. and Canada). Fax: 314-447-8029. E-mail: journals customerservice-usa@elsevier.com (for print support); journalsonlinesupport-usa@elsevier.com (for online support).**

Reprints. For copies of 100 or more, of articles in this publication, please contact the Commercial Reprints Department, Elsevier Inc., 360 Park Avenue South, New York, NY 10010-1710. Tel.: 212-633-3874; Fax: 212-633-3820; Email: reprints@elsevier.com.

Oral and Maxillofacial Surgery Clinics of North America is covered in *MEDLINE/PubMed* (*Index Medicus*), *Science Citation Index Expanded (SciSearch®), Journal Citation Reports/Science Edition,* and *Current Contents®/Clinical Medicine.*

Contributors

CONSULTING EDITOR

RICHARD H. HAUG, DDS
Professor and Chief, Oral Maxillofacial Surgery, Carolinas Medical Center, Charlotte, North Carolina

EDITORS

JEFFREY D. BENNETT, DMD
Associate Professor, Oral and Maxillofacial Surgery; Chief, Division of Oral and Maxillofacial Surgery, Roudebush VA Medical Center; Clinical Professor, Department of Oral and Maxillofacial Surgery, Indiana University, Indianapolis, Indiana

ELIE M. FERNEINI, DMD, MD, MHS, MBA, FACS
Private Practice, Greater Waterbury OMS; Medical Director, Beau Visage Med Spa, Cheshire, Connecticut; Assistant Clinical Professor, Division of Oral and Maxillofacial Surgery, Department of Craniofacial Sciences, University of Connecticut, Farmington, Connecticut

AUTHORS

CHASE L. ANDREASON, DMD
Department of Oral Surgery and Hospital Dentistry, Indiana University School of Dentistry, Indianapolis, Indiana

JEFFREY D. BENNETT, DMD
Associate Professor, Oral and Maxillofacial Surgery; Chief, Division of Oral and Maxillofacial Surgery, Roudebush VA Medical Center; Clinical Professor, Department of Oral and Maxillofacial Surgery, Indiana University, Indianapolis, Indiana

ROBERT BONA, MD, FACP
Professor of Medical Sciences, Frank H. Netter School of Medicine, Quinnipiac University, Hamden, Connecticut

EHLIE K. BRUNO, DDS
OMFS Resident, Indiana University, Indianapolis, Indiana

ANTOINE M. FERNEINI, MD, FACS
Section Chief, Division of Vascular Surgery, Yale-New Haven Hospital/St. Raphael Campus, New Haven, Connecticut; Private Practice, Connecticut Vascular Center, PC, North Haven, Connecticut

ELIE M. FERNEINI, DMD, MD, MHS, MBA, FACS
Private Practice, Greater Waterbury OMS; Medical Director, Beau Visage Med Spa, Cheshire, Connecticut; Assistant Clinical Professor, Division of Oral and Maxillofacial Surgery, Department of Craniofacial Sciences, University of Connecticut, Farmington, Connecticut

LAURA GART, DMD
Oral and Maxillofacial Surgery Resident, Division of Oral and Maxillofacial Surgery, Yale-New Haven Hospital, New Haven, Connecticut

ANDRE E. GHANTOUS, MD, FACC
Assistant Clinical Professor, Division of Cardiology, Department of Medicine, Yale University School of Medicine, New Haven, Connecticut

ARMAN G. HAGHIGHI, DDS
Resident, Department of Oral and Maxillofacial Surgery, Indiana University, Indianapolis, Indiana

THOMAS M. HALASZYNSKI, DMD, MD, MBA
Associate Professor of Anesthesiology, Department of Anesthesiology, Yale University School of Medicine, New Haven, Connecticut

REGINA L. LANDESBERG, DMD, PhD
Private Practice, Greater Waterbury OMS, Waterbury, Connecticut

LISAMARIE DI PASQUALE, DDS, MD
Resident, Division of Oral and Maxillofacial Surgery, Department of Craniofacial Sciences, University of Connecticut, Farmington, Connecticut

TIMOTHY H. POHLMAN, MD, FACS
Trauma Services, Division of General Surgery, Department of Surgery, Methodist Hospital, Indiana University Health, Indianapolis, Indiana

JULIE ANN SMITH, DDS, MD, MCR
Oral and Maxillofacial Surgeon, Willamette Dental Group; Affiliate Associate Professor, Oregon Health and Science University, Portland, Oregon

MARTIN B. STEED, DDS
Associate Professor and Chair, Department of Oral and Maxillofacial Surgery, Medical University of South Carolina, Charleston, South Carolina

MATTHEW T. SWANSON, DDS
Department of Oral and Maxillofacial Surgery, Chief Resident, Medical University of South Carolina, Charleston, South Carolina

REBECCA G. FINDER, PharmD, BCPS
Resident, Critical Care Pharmacy, Indiana University Health, Indianapolis, Indiana

PATRICK J. VEZEAU, DDS, MS
Oral Surgery and Implant Specialists, Private Practice, Dakota Dunes, South Dakota

Contents

Oral healthcare providers are concerned with best practice management of patients prescribed coagulation-altering therapy during the perioperative/periprocedural periods for dental and oral surgery interventions. Recommendations can be based on medication pharmacology, coagulation factor levels/deficiencies, degree of clinical invasiveness, and patient comorbidities. Caution must always be used with concurrent use of medications that can affect different components of the clotting mechanisms and prompt diagnosis along with necessary intervention may be needed to optimize outcome. However, evidence-based data on management of anticoagulants during interventions is lacking. Therefore, clinical understanding and judgment are needed along with appropriate guidelines matching patient- and intervention-specific recommendations.

There are multiple systemic diseases that have an impact on coagulation, of which oral and maxillofacial surgeons must be cognizant. Recent evidence has supported the potential for both hypocoagulable and hypercoagulable states in patients with liver and kidney disease with an even less understood impact on prolonged bleeding in the oral cavity. These systemic diseases are not limited to diseases affecting the liver, kidney, and bone marrow; however, these diseases are common among the patient population and surgeons must be capable of making appropriate judgment and modifying care appropriately.

Platelet abnormalities result from a wide range of congenital and acquired conditions, which may be known or unknown to patients presenting for oral maxillofacial surgery. It is critical to obtain a thorough history, including discussion of any episodes of bleeding or easy bruising, to potentially discern patients with an underlying platelet disorder. If patients indicate a positive history, preoperative laboratory studies are indicated, with potential referral or consultation with a hematologist. Appropriate preoperative planning may reduce the risk of bleeding associated with platelet dysfunction, potentially avoiding serious perioperative and postoperative complications.

Hemophilia will be encountered in the oral and maxillofacial surgeon's office. A thorough understanding of hemophilia is necessary to safely care for these patients. One must understand the severity of the patient's hemophilia as well as whether or not inhibitors are present. The patient's surgical management will be influenced by these two factors. In addition to the possible need to transfuse factors or desmopressin, special care must be taken perioperatively to avoid bleeding complications. This article reviews the overall management of hemophilia A and B as well as the specific perioperative management of these patients.

Thrombophilia or hypercoagulable conditions can be thought of as either inherited or acquired. The inherited disorders include deficiencies of antithrombin, protein C, or protein S or the common disorders of factor V Leiden and prothrombin G20210A gene mutation. All these disorders are inherited as autosomal dominant and predispose individuals primarily to venous thrombosis. Acquired thrombophilic conditions are seen in individuals with cancer, phospholipid antibodies, and a whole host of other conditions that alter endothelial function, change blood levels of coagulant or anticoagulant proteins, activate platelets, or have other effects on coagulation proteins, platelet function, or the endothelium.

Most patients with coronary artery disease and peripheral vascular disease are on long-term antiplatelet therapy and dual therapy. Achieving a balance between ischemic and bleeding risk remains an important factor in managing patients on antiplatelet therapy. For most outpatient surgical procedures, maintenance and continuation of this therapy are recommended. Consultation with the patient's cardiologist, physician, and/or vascular surgeon is always recommended before interrupting or withholding this treatment modality.

For the oral and maxillofacial surgeon, many patients will be on heparin products during surgery. So far, there is no standardized approach to treating anticoagulated patients during oral and maxillofacial surgical procedures. When a patient is on heparin therapy, heparin may be stopped 4 to 6 hours before surgery and resumed once hemostasis is achieved, usually within 24 hours. If low-molecular-weight heparin is administered, the treatment is generally stopped at least 12 hours before surgery and then resumed in a similar fashion. Local measures are generally enough to provide adequate hemostasis.

The new direct oral anticoagulants-dabigatran etexilate, rivaroxaban, and apixaban-have predictable pharmacokinetic and pharmacodynamic profiles and are alternatives to warfarin. However, many surgeons are wary of these drugs, as there is limited evidence on how to manage bleeding in patients taking them, and only recently has a specific antidote been developed to reverse their anticoagulant effect. Management of the newer agents requires careful adherence to primary measures of bleeding care, knowledge of their mechanism of action, and familiarity with the unapproved and untested reversal strategies that may be required in patients with life-threatening bleeding.

Hemostasis is a key step in safe and predictable surgery. Knowledge of normal blood clotting mechanisms and abnormal diathesis is necessary to anticipate potential problems during and after surgery. As an adjunct to bleeding control, topical hemostatic agents have long been used in all surgical disciplines. This article provides a brief review of hemostasis and a topical summary of different classes of topical hemostatic agents useful to oral and maxillofacial surgery, including indications and potential complications/side effects. This rapidly evolving field promises to yield future agents with increased efficacy, cost efficiency, and decreased complications.

Endovascular techniques are essential for controlling acute head and neck bleeding that cannot be controlled by local or systemic measures. Detailed knowledge of the head and neck vascular anatomy, advances in catheterization techniques, and the availability of new embolic materials have improved the safety, efficacy, and predictability of these procedures. To improve patient safety, the oral and maxillofacial surgeon must be familiar with these techniques.

Blood products are routinely used to manage various coagulation and hematological disorders. However, there is a debate in the medical literature concerning the appropriate use of blood and blood products. Oral and maxillofacial surgeons must have a basic knowledge and understanding of the various available products. A consultation with each patient's hematologist is always advised in order to decrease the risk of adverse events and improve the patient's safety.

The recognition and management of massive blood loss as a consequence of severe facial trauma or as a complication of complex oral and maxillofacial procedures pose formidable challenges. A patient who has lost substantial amounts of blood may still present in a deceptive clinical state that suggests stability, although oxygen delivery to tissue is severely compromised. Furthermore, hemorrhagic shock may be compounded by specific hemostatic disorders induced by trauma and several

Contents

extreme homeostatic imbalances that often appear during resuscitation. We review salient clinical features of these hemorrhage-induced processes and describe recent advances in damage control resuscitation for management of them.

ORAL AND MAXILLOFACIAL SURGERY CLINICS OF NORTH AMERICA

Erratum

In the August 2016 issue (Volume 28, number 3), for the article "Painful Traumatic Trigeminal Neuropathy," all of the authors' names were incorrectly cited. The correct author names should be Rafael Benoliel, Sorin Teich, and Eli Eliav, and the correct article reference is Benoliel R, Teich ST, Eliav E. Painful Traumatic Trigeminal Neuropathy. Oral Maxillofac Surg Clin North Am 2016;28(3):371-380.

Oral Maxillofacial Surg Clin N Am 28 (2016) xi
http://dx.doi.org/10.1016/j.coms.2016.08.002

Preface

Coagulopathy Management: The Balance Between Thromboembolism and Hemorrhage

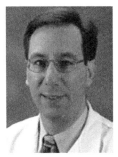

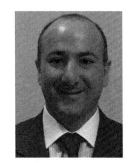

Jeffrey D. Bennett, DMD   Elie M. Ferneini, DMD, MD, MHS, MBA, FACS

Editors

It ought … to be understood that no one can be a good physician who has no idea of surgical operations, and that a surgeon is nothing if ignorant of medicine. In a word, one must be familiar with both departments of medicine.
— *Guido Lanfranchi*

A basic tenet of surgery is understanding hemostasis. The surgeon must be knowledgeable with disease processes associated with abnormal hemostasis, be able to recognize signs and symptoms identifying potential abnormal hemostasis, be familiar with the growing list of coagulation-altering therapy, and be up-to-date with management protocols to optimize patient care.

This issue is devoted to the management of the patients with a congenital or a therapeutic coagulopathy. The authors selected for this issue are recognized experts in their specialty, and they provide the most current and up-to-date data on the medical and surgical management of these patients.

As oral and maxillofacial surgeons, we are faced with medically compromised patients with systemic diseases, which alter hemostasis, and those who are therapeutically taking coagulation-altering therapy on a daily basis. In the last 20 years, prophylactic as well as therapeutic use of coagulation-altering therapy has been increasing due to the rise in prevalence of coronary artery disease, atrial fibrillation, vascular disease, thromboembolic events, and other risk factors of our aging US population. Careful management of the patient with risk for altered hemostasis or taking anticoagulant drugs in the perioperative period is essential in treating our surgical patients. Many surgeons may not have any established perioperative management guidelines.

The patient with a congenital or therapeutic coagulopathy requires a surgeon who is "familiar with both departments of medicine." The surgeon must employ both his or her medical knowledge and surgical skill to achieve a balance between thromboembolism and perioperative bleeding. Many of these patients may require interdisciplinary management by a team of different medical and surgical specialties. Many medical specialists may not understand the scope and intricacies of the various oral and maxillofacial surgical procedures. There is a lack of knowledge of the risk of

Oral Maxillofacial Surg Clin N Am 28 (2016) xiii–xiv
http://dx.doi.org/10.1016/j.coms.2016.08.001
1042-3699/16/© 2016 Published by Elsevier Inc.

hemorrhage or the ability to locally achieve hemostasis, which may result in an inappropriate recommendation. It is, therefore, important that we seek input and assistance when such is required but alternatively are neither passive nor silent with sharing our knowledge to ensure optimal patient management.

Jeffrey D. Bennett, DMD
Oral and Maxillofacial Surgery Section
Roudebush VA Medical Center
Oral and Maxillofacial Surgery
Indiana University
Indianapolis, IN, USA

Elie M. Ferneini, DMD, MD, MHS, MBA, FACS
Greater Waterbury OMS
Beau Visage Med Spa
435 Highland Avenue, Suite 100
Cheshire, CT 06410, USA

Division of Oral and Maxillofacial Surgery
Department of Craniofacial Sciences
University of Connecticut
263 Farmington Avenue
Farmington, CT 06030, USA

E-mail addresses:
jb2omfs@gmail.com (J.D. Bennett)
eferneini@yahoo.com (E.M. Ferneini)

Administration of Coagulation-Altering Therapy in the Patient Presenting for Oral Health and Maxillofacial Surgery

Thomas M. Halaszynski, DMD, MD, MBA

KEYWORDS

- Hemostasis/coagulation • Anticoagulation therapy • Oral and maxillofacial surgery
- Specialty-society anticoagulation guidelines and recommendations • Dual-anticoagulation therapy
- www.WarfarinDosing.org

KEY POINTS

- Evidence-based data on management of anticoagulation therapy during oral and maxillofacial surgery/interventions are lacking.
- Clinical understanding and judgment are needed along with the most appropriate guidelines matching patient- and intervention-specific recommendations.
- To reduce serious dysfunction from hemorrhagic complications, one should implement "general surgery" patient recommendations.
- It is important to follow consensus statements of recognized experts in anticoagulation, review the pharmacology of medication package inserts, and request a hematology consult when necessary.
- The oral surgeon should understand risk factors for bleeding and how to treat bleeding complications.

INTRODUCTION

Prophylactic and therapeutic use of coagulation-altering therapy has been increasing owing to the increase in prevalence of coronary artery disease, atrial fibrillation (AF), and other risk factors of the aging US population.[1] As a result, several commonly used anticoagulants being prescribed along with action plans for use during the perioperative period and in outpatient settings with emphasis on management and considerations for appropriate decision-making alternatives are discussed herein. It is also intended to assist oral and dental health care providers in periprocedural anticoagulation management in the general patient population. However, it remains necessary that patient-specific evaluation of bleeding risks associated with the specific planned procedure as well as thromboembolic risks associated with any underlying disease that requires anticoagulation is investigated and understood. Deciding on patient-specific management plans (including holding therapy) should usually be made in consultation with the prescribing physician and the oral health care specialist performing the procedure, and then communicated directly to the patient. The management of patients receiving

Disclosure: This article has no any commercial or financial conflicts of interest and has received no support from external funding sources.
Department of Anesthesiology, Yale University School of Medicine, 333 Cedar Street, TMP 3 Library, New Haven, CT 203 785-2804, USA
E-mail address: thomas.halaszynski@yale.edu

Oral Maxillofacial Surg Clin N Am 28 (2016) 443–460
http://dx.doi.org/10.1016/j.coms.2016.06.005

coagulation-altering medications (**Box 1**) recommends against concurrent use of medications (aspirin and other nonsteroidal antiinflammatory drugs) that affect other components of the clotting mechanism and can increase the risk(s) of bleeding complications.[2–4] Therefore, appropriate perioperative and periprocedural judgment is needed when making decisions about coagulation-altering therapy (continue, discontinue, or consider bridge therapy) and when to resume anticoagulation, in addition to recommendations regarding the time points when these events should occur.[5]

The incidence of hemorrhagic complications associated with performing oral and maxillofacial surgery/interventions in the patient receiving coagulation-altering therapy is unknown. Patient safety considerations defy prospective randomized study, and there is no proven or current laboratory model to implement. As a result, maxillofacial surgeons usually follow recommendations for general surgery patients. In addition, what has been portrayed in this article in investigation of the current dental and medical literature based on consensus statements representing the collective experiences of recognized experts in anticoagulation, case reports, clinical series, pharmacology, hematology, and risk factors for bleeding. Also summarized and adapted here in this article, in response to dental and oral health patient safety issues, are specialty society consensus conference guidelines and suggestions for the anticoagulated patient.[2–4,6–10] These practice guidelines or recommendations that summarize evidence-based reviews from the literature were compiled and discussed herein with a relatively conservative approach toward managing oral and maxillofacial surgery along with more routine dental interventions in patients on coagulation-altering medications. There is a lack of evidence-based guidelines for safely managing oral and maxillofacial patients taking anticoagulation medications; therefore, summary information from medical and dental specialty sources has been performed and divided into perioperative and periprocedural sections.

Box 1
Classes of hemostasis-altering medications

Herbal medications

- Garlic
- Ginkgo
- Ginseng

Antiplatelet medications

- Aspirin
- Nonsteroidal antiinflammatory drugs
- Thienopyridine derivatives (ticlopidine, clopidogrel)
- Platelet glycoprotein IIb/IIIa inhibitors (GPIIb/IIIa receptor antagonists)

Unfractionated heparin intravenous and subcutaneous

Low-molecular-weight heparin

Vitamin K antagonists: warfarin

Thrombin (factor IIa) inhibitors

- Desirudin
- Lepirudin
- Bivalirudin
- Argatroban

Factor Xa inhibitors

- Fondaparinux
- Rivaroxaban
- Apixaban
- Edoxaban

Thrombolytic and Fibrinolysis Medications

- Tissue plasminogen activator
- Streptokinase
- Urokinase
- Anistreplase

HERBAL MEDICATIONS AND ANTIPLATELET DRUGS

Many patients use herbal medications with potential for complications because of polypharmacy and physiologic alterations. Some complications include bleeding from garlic, ginkgo, and ginseng, along with the potential interaction between ginseng and warfarin. It remains important to be familiar with literature on herbals secondary to new discoveries about effects in humans. However, herbal medications, when administered independent to other coagulation-altering therapy is not a contraindication to planned interventions/surgery.

Aspirin and other nonsteroidal antiinflammatory drugs, when administered alone during the perioperative/periprocedural period, are not considered a contraindication. In patients on combination therapy with medications affecting more than 1 coagulation mechanism, clinicians should be cautious about increased risks of bleeding.[11,12] Cyclooxygenase-2 inhibitors have shown minimal effect on platelet function, are considered safe for patients, and are without additive effects in the presence of anticoagulation therapy.[2]

Antiplatelet medications including thienopyridine derivatives and platelet glycoprotein (GP) IIb/IIIa antagonists have diverse pharmacologic effects on coagulation and platelet function. Such differences are challenging, because there are no acceptable tests to guide therapy. Assessment should search for considerations that contribute to altered coagulation (bruising easily, excessive bleeding, female sex with advanced age), but risks with ticlopidine/clopidogrel and the GPIIb/IIIa antagonists remain unknown. Therefore, management is based on labeling, surgical reviews, invasiveness of surgery/intervention, bleeding risks, and usually includes (1) time between discontinuation of therapy is 14 days for ticlopidine and 5 to 7 days for clopidogrel, (2) if proceeding (especially with invasive interventions) before completing suggested time interval(s), then normalization of platelet function should be demonstrated, and (3) platelet GPIIb/IIIa inhibitors exert effect on platelet aggregation and time to normal platelet aggregation is 24 to 48 hours for abciximab and 4 to 8 hours for eptifibatide and tirofiban after discontinuation.[13] GPIIb/IIIa antagonists are typically contraindicated within 4 weeks of surgery.

THROMBIN INHIBITORS

Thrombin inhibitors medications interrupt the proteolysis properties of thrombin. Unlike heparin, thrombin inhibitors influence fibrin formation and inactivate fibrin already bound to thrombin (inhibiting further thrombus formation). These medications lack an antidote, but the hirudins and argatroban can be removed with dialysis.

Hirudins: Desirudin, Lepirudin, and Bivalirudin

These are direct thrombin inhibitors and indicated for thromboprophylaxis (desirudin), prevention of deep vein thrombosis (DVT) and pulmonary embolism (PE) after hip replacement for example,[14] and DVT treatment (lepirudin) in patients with heparin-induced thrombocytopenia (HIT).[15] They have an elimination half-life of 30 minutes to 3 hours, can accumulate with renal insufficiency, and should be monitored using activated partial thromboplastin time (aPTT) or ecarin clotting time (which is a more specific). Prolonged aPTT is required for effective thromboprophylaxis, and there is still a prolonged aPTT 8 hours after subcutaneous (SC) administration of low-dose hirudins. Lepirudin has been associated with antibody formation (incidence of 40%), delayed elimination, unpredictable and prolonged activity, as well as association with bleeding and anaphylaxis.[16]

Owing to lack of information and application(s) of these agents, no statement(s) regarding risk and patient management can be made (HIT patients typically need therapeutic levels of anticoagulation making them poor candidates for invasive procedures). Administration of thrombin inhibitors in combination with other antithrombotic agents should always be avoided, and under emergency circumstances, it is recommended to wait a minimum of 8 to 10 hours after the last dose when possible, along with evidence of normal aPTT or ecarin clotting time. Secondary to bleeding concerns, the trend with these thrombin inhibitors has been to replace them with factor Xa inhibitors (ie, fondaparinux for DVT prophylaxis or argatroban for acute HIT).

Argatroban

Argatroban is administered intravenously, reversible, and a direct thrombin inhibitor approved for management of acute HIT (type II). Advantages over other thrombin inhibitors include its elimination through the liver (indication in compromising renal dysfunction) and short half-life (35–40 min) that reveals normalization of aPTT in 2 to 4 hours after discontinuation. Dose reduction should be considered in the critically ill, and those with heart failure or impaired hepatic function.

THROMBOLYTICS AND FIBRINOLYTICS

These agents dissolve clot(s) secondary to the action of plasmin. The plasminogen activators streptokinase and urokinase dissolve thrombus and influence plasminogen, leading to decreased levels of plasminogen and fibrin. Thrombolytic therapy will maximally depress fibrinogen and plasminogen 5 hours after therapy and remain depressed for 27 hours.[17] Original recommendations to initiate thrombolytic therapy was contraindicated within 10 days after surgery, but in a recent consensus statement it was reduced to 2-day minimum.[2] The 2-day minimum is based on prolonged plasminogen depression of 27 hours. Definitive data are not available on when to discontinue these agents and the safe time to proceed with invasive interventions as clots are not stable for 10 days after thrombolytic therapy.[2] However, performing superficial procedures (bleeding easily managed) earlier than 10 days can be evaluated with caution on an individual basis weighing the risk-to-benefit ratio.

ANTICOAGULANTS
Unfractionated Heparin

- Activates antithrombin III.
- Therapeutic levels achieved prolongation of aPTT of 2 to 3 times,
- Anti–factor Xa levels between 0.3 and 0.7 U/mL.

Heparin-treated patients who develop serious bleeding can be given protamine sulfate to neutralize heparin using 1 mg of protamine to neutralize 100 U of heparin. A serious side effect of heparin includes thrombocytopenia (most serious form being HIT thrombosis syndrome or HIT-type 2). HIT type 1 (not immune mediated) can result in a mild decrease in platelet count, but does not usually involve significant bleeding risks. However, patients with HIT type 2 (immune mediated) can have dangerously low platelet counts that occur 5 to 14 days after initiating heparin therapy.[18] There are also exceptions in which HIT type 2 can occur either earlier or later than the described time frame.[18]

Low-Molecular-Weight Heparin

- Activates antithrombin III and subsequently inhibits factor Xa.
- Does not usually require coagulation test monitoring.

Low-molecular-weight heparin (LMWH) has been used increasingly to replace heparin administration and is usually administered SC. Enoxaparin (Lovenox) and dalteparin (Fragmin) have several advantages compared with heparin, such as dose-independent clearance, more predictable anticoagulant response, improved bioavailability after SC injection, and lower risks of osteoporosis and HIT.[19] Coagulation test monitoring, if necessary, can use anti–factor Xa level measuring, because there is little to no effect of LMWH on the aPTT. Therapeutic anti–factor Xa levels range from 0.5 to 1.2 U/mL and levels of 0.2 to 0.5 U/mL are desirable for prophylactic prescribing.[20] LMWH monitoring is indicated in those with renal insufficiency, but not typically performed in obese patients.[21] Protamine will incompletely neutralize the anticoagulant activity of this medication because it only binds to the longer chains of LMWH.

Fondaparinux (Arixtra)

- Indicated for thromboprophylaxis.
- Exerts effect through factor Xa inhibition.

Fondaparinux used as an alternative to heparin or LMWH for initial treatment in those with established venous thromboembolism (VTE). With no binding to endothelial cells or plasma proteins, its clearance is dose independent and plasma half-life is 17 hours.[19] Because this medication is cleared unchanged by the kidneys, it can be considered as contraindicated in patients with renal insufficiency.

Warfarin (Coumadin, Jantoven, Marevan)

- Interferes with synthesis of vitamin K–dependent clotting proteins (factors II, VII, IX, and X).
- Metabolized in the liver (cytochrome P450) system; drugs that induce or inhibit cytochrome P450 can alter its metabolism.
- Administered in doses to achieve international normalized ratio (INR) of 2.0 to 3.0 for most clinical indications (exception in patients with mechanical mitral heart valves; an higher INR [2.5–3.5] is recommended).

Because of the delay in achieving antithrombotic effects, initial therapy with warfarin is combined with concomitant administration of a more rapidly acting parenteral anticoagulant (heparin, LMWH, or fondaparinux). Warfarin is absorbed rapidly from the gastrointestinal tract and levels of warfarin in the blood peak about 90 minutes after drug administration with a plasma half-life of 36 to 42 hours.[22]

The newer oral anticoagulants (NOACs) available in the United States include dabigatran (direct thrombin inhibitor), and several anti–factor Xa agents (such as rivaroxaban, apixaban, and edoxaban; **Table 1**). The NOACs have a rapid onset of action and peak anticoagulant effect achieved within 2 to 3 hours that could potentially reduce any need for temporary parenteral anticoagulation.

Dabigatran (Pradaxa)

- Oral direct thrombin inhibitor (half-life 12–14 hours).
- Maximum anticoagulantion within 2 to 3 hours.

Unchanged renal excretion of dabigatran is the predominant elimination pathway, with drug clearance being longer in older adults and those with reduced renal function. Routine monitoring of coagulation is not typically used for patients taking dabigatran (the INR should not be used to monitor therapy).[23]

Rivaroxaban (Xarelto)

- Oral direct factor Xa inhibitor (bioavailability of 80% and half-life 7–11 hours).
- Peak plasma concentrations within 2.5 to 4 hours.

Rivaroxaban is not recommended in patients with renal insufficiency or those with significant hepatic impairment (can prolong half-life).[22]

Table 1
Oral anticoagulants: properties and indications

Drug	Mechanism	Half-Life (h)	Time to Peak Serum Level (h)	Metabolism	Indications
Warfarin	Vitamin K antagonist	36–42	1.5	Hepatic, oxidative metabolism	DVT/PE treatment DVT prophylaxis AF (valvular and nonvalvular)
Rivaroxaban	Factor Xa inhibitor	7–11	2–4	33% renal (remainder metabolized to inactive molecules and eliminated in the feces and urine)	DVT prophylaxis after knee/hip surgery DVT/PE treatment Nonvalvular AF
Apixaban	Factor Xa inhibitor	8–15	3–4	25% renal	DVT prophylaxis after knee/hip surgery DVT/PE treatment Nonvalvular AF
Edoxaban	Factor Xa inhibitor	9–10	1–2	35% renal	DVT/PE treatment Nonvalvular AF
Dabigatran	Direct thrombin inhibitor	10–14	1.5	80% renal elimination	DVT/PE treatment Nonvalvular AF

Abbreviations: AT, atrial fibrillation; DVT, deep venous thrombosis; PE, pulmonary embolism.

Apixaban (Eliquis)

- Oral direct and selective inhibitor of factor Xa.
- Approved for AF and treatment of VTE.
- Peak plasma concentrations approximately 3 hours (half-life of 8–15 hours).

It is mostly eliminated through hepatic metabolism and fecal route with approximately 25% excreted renally.[24]

Edoxaban (Savaysa)

- Direct factor Xa inhibitor.
- Peak plasma concentration in 1 to 2 hours.
- Half-life of 9 to 10 hours.

Edoxaban is indicated for extended treatment of DVT and PE after 5 to 10 days of initial therapy with a parenteral anticoagulant. This medication should not be used in patients with a creatinine clearance of greater than 95 mL/min that can led to decreased efficacy. It also carries an increased risk of ischemic stroke compared with warfarin. Approximately 50% of the drug is excreted renally with the remainder eliminated through metabolism and biliary excretion.[25]

PERIOPERATIVE MANAGEMENT OF COAGULATION-ALTERING THERAPY

Clinicians must always assess the risk(s) versus benefits of thrombosis associated with discontinuing any antithrombotic agent and balance that against potential bleeding risk(s) that could be inherent to routine oral health interventions, invasive procedures or maxillofacial surgery. For example, management of patients taking warfarin can often differ from those on NOACs such that: warfarin is usually discontinued 5 to 7 days before invasive surgery to allow for normalization of the INR, but thrombotic risk(s) can necessitate an assessment of whether a form of "bridging" therapy (using short-acting parenteral medications such as LMWH or UFH) should be considered during this time period (time between discontinuing warfarin and time of the clinical intervention). In contrast, given the short half-life of NOACs, these medications can be stopped within a shorter time period before any planned clinical procedure or surgical intervention without a need for a bridging agent. However, additional considerations need to be extended to perioperative management of patients prescribed with both vitamin K antagonists and NOACs by following a stepwise approach similar to the 4 steps described.

Step 1: Assessment of bleeding risks by addressing whether the anticoagulant needs to be stopped for the proposed procedure/surgery or can the procedure be performed while the patient is on anticoagulation medication;
Step 2: Deciding on the duration of preoperative interruption of any particular antithrombotic agent;

Step 3: Defining thrombotic risks by addressing what is the patient's risk of suffering a thromboembolic event owing to perioperative interruption of anticoagulation; and

Step 4: Consideration of any need for bridging therapy (ie, for those prescribed warfarin if the patient is at high risk of a thromboembolic event owing to perioperative interruption of anticoagulation).

Perioperative Management of Patients on Warfarin

Step 1: assessing the bleeding risk

Assessment of perioperative bleeding risk(s) involves an understanding of the patient's comorbidities and invasive nature of any proposed intervention/procedure. Although no clear predictors of bleeding risk have been validated during the perioperative period, there is evidence linking active cancer, thrombocytopenia (platelets < 150,000), presence of a mechanical mitral valve or a history of bleeding to an increased risk of invasive oral health care interventions and perioperative bleeding.[26,27] Although developed for nonoperative and nonprocedural situations and to facilitate decisions of whether to start anticoagulation in patients with AF, the HAS-BLED score takes into account a history of *h*ypertension, *a*bnormal renal/liver function, *s*troke, *b*leeding history or predisposition toward bleeding, *l*abile INR values, the *e*lderly (>65 years of age), and concomitant use of *d*rugs/alcohol.[28,29] In addition, the HAS-BLED score has also been found to be useful in assessing potential of bleeding risk if bridging therapy is being considered.[30]

Current evidence supports that in patients prescribed with warfarin who are scheduled for procedures with low risks of bleeding that they can be performed without interruption of such therapy and that an INR of 2.5 or less can be accepted as safe.[31,32] For example, minor dermatologic procedures such as removal of squamous cell and basal cell carcinomas or actinic keratosis can be safely performed with higher INR values (<3.5).[33] Patients undergoing more routine dental procedures, including extractions, biopsies, and periodontal surgeries can continue their warfarin perioperatively as long as the INR is less than 4.[10,34] Injections can also be performed without discontinuing warfarin therapy.[3]

Step 2: deciding on the duration of preoperative interruption of any particular antithrombotic agent

Discontinuing warfarin therapy should be considered before surgeries that carry an intermediate to high risk of bleeding (**Table 2**) in which warfarin is stopped 5 days before the proposed procedure for the INR to normalize before the intervention.[3] The rate of decline or normalization of the INR after warfarin discontinuation is related to starting INR values rather than the prescribed dosage of the medication.[35] Patients maintained at higher INR values (3–4) as well as the elderly often require a longer interruption period.[36] Although normal hemostasis has been demonstrated for INR levels between 1 and 2 (sufficient for adequate hemostasis respectively corresponding with 100% and 30% clotting factor activity), an INR of less than 1.5 can be accepted for most procedures.[3,27,31] Patients scheduled for very high-risk surgical procedures require documentation of a normal INR on the day of the anticipated intervention.[4,10,32] However, despite holding warfarin for 5 to 7 days, it is still possible that the INR does not fall within the reference range on the day of surgery and administering a small dose of oral vitamin K (1–2.5 mg), preferably the day before any planned procedure if the INR is 1.4–1.9) could be beneficial.[37]

Special considerations for high-risk bleeding procedures Various high-risk bleeding procedures can be performed while continuing warfarin therapy, but cautious considerations must be extended. For example, the recommendation is to continue warfarin aiming for an INR between 2 and 3 rather then use bridging therapy that can increase the risk of periprocedural stoke and bleeding owing to LMWH.[38,39] Soft tissue intercavity and intracavity interventions can also be performed without interruption of warfarin administration as bridging therapy can lead to a higher risk of pocket hematoma formation.[40,41]

Step 3: defining the thrombotic risk and considerations for bridging

The 2012 American College of Chest Physicians Evidence-Based Clinical Practice Guidelines, 9th edition, on Perioperative management of antithrombotic therapy (2012 ACCP guidelines) provides a framework for managing patients on anticoagulation who are to undergo a wide spectrum of elective surgical interventions.[3] The take-home message of these guidelines is evidenced by the classification of patients prescribed warfarin for AF, mechanical valves or VTE/PE according to their thrombotic risk (**Table 3**). Patients in the high-risk category have an annual risk of thrombosis of greater than 10%, patients in the moderate risk category 5% to 10% risk of thrombosis, and patients in the low-risk category, a risk of thrombosis of less than 5%.[2,3]

Warfarin for atrial fibrillation AF is a commonly encountered cardiac arrhythmia in the elderly

Table 2
Bleeding risk based on the procedure

Procedure	Low Risk Bleeding (<1.5%)	High Risk Bleeding (>1.5%, or in Vulnerable Areas)
Anesthesiology	Endotracheal intubation	—
Dental	Tooth extraction Endodontic procedures (root canal)	Reconstructive procedures
Dermatology	Minor skin procedures (excision of basal and squamous cell cancers, nevi, actinic keratoses, premalignant lesions)	Major procedures (wide excision of melanoma)
General surgery	Suture of superficial wounds	Major tissue injury Exploration
Interventional radiology	Simple catheter exchange in well-formed, nonvascular tracts Placement of small-caliber drains Peripheral catheter placement, nontunneled catheter (peripherally inserted central catheter) placement Inferior vena cava filter placement Temporary dialysis catheter placement	Chest tube placement Aggressive manipulation of drains or dilation of tracts Hickman and tunneled dialysis catheter placement
Intravascular procedures	Venous access	Arterial puncture
Ophthalmology	—	Periorbital surgery
Otolaryngologic surgery	Fiberoptic laryngoscopy or nasopharyngoscopy, sinus endoscopy Fine-needle aspiration Vocal cord injection	Any sinus surgery Biopsy or removal of nasal polyps Septoplasty Turbinate cautery
Plastic surgery	Injection therapy	Reconstruction

Adapted from Baron TH, Kamath PS, McBane RD. Management of antithrombotic therapy in patients undergoing invasive procedures. N Engl J Med 2013;368(22):2118; with permission.

population with an annual increased risk of stroke of 5% to 8% in the absence of anticoagulation. The stroke risk from AF decreases to 1.6% in patients who are treated with warfarin.[42] Concern for risks of stroke during interruption of anticoagulation therapy can be estimated using the CHADS2 (Congestive heart failure, Hypertension, Age [>65 = 1 point; >75 = 2 points], Diabetes, and Stroke/transient ischemic attack) and CHA2DS2-VASc (Congestive heart failure, Hypertension, Age > 75 years, Diabetes, and Stroke/transient ischemic attack, Vascular disease, Age 65-74 years, Sex category) scores (it should be noted that these parameters have not been validated in the perioperative setting; **Table 4**). In addition, surgical trauma often induces a proinflammatory/prothrombotic state that can result in an increased risk of stroke in the presence of AF.[43]

The CHA2DS2-VASc model is more discriminating than the CHADS2 score in identifying low-risk patients (CHA2DS2-VASc of 0) as well as classifying more accurately the intermediate risk patient population.[44] However, although the CHA2DS2-VASc can more accurately lead to a decision of whether to place patients with AF

on anticoagulation therapy, the CHADS2 score can more precisely determine whether bridging therapy needs to be initiated in the event anticoagulation interruption is considered for those taking warfarin. Therefore, based on the 2012 ACCP guidelines, patients with CHADS2 scores of 0 to 2 do not require bridging therapy, but patients with CHADS2 scores of 5 to 6 can benefit from initiating anticoagulation bridging therapy. For patients with intermediate CHADS2 scores of 3 to 4, any decision to start bridging therapy should be at the discretion of the patient's cardiologist.[3] However, more recent literature suggests bridging for patients with AF and a CHA2DS2-VASc score of 2 or higher, even though the CHADS2 score was found to predict postoperative stroke.[45]

Consideration of benefits associated with bridging therapy should always be weighed against the increased risk of perioperative bleeding, challenging the antithrombotic benefit of bridging. A metaanalysis involving 34 studies described a 13% to 15% risk for perioperative bleeding and 3% to 4% increased risk for major bleeding, with no evidence of decreased risk for

Table 3
Thromboembolic risk based on indication for warfarin

Indication for Warfarin	Low Risk	Moderate Risk	High Risk
AF	CHA2DS2-VASc score of 2–3 or CHADS2 score of 0–2 (assuming no prior stroke or transient ischemic attack)	CHA2DS2-VASc score of 4–5 or CHADS2 score of 3–4	CHA2DS2-VASc score of ≥6 or CHADS2 score of 5–6 Recent (within 3 mo) stroke or transient ischemic attack Rheumatic valvular heart disease
Mechanical heart valve	Bileaflet aortic valve prosthesis without AF, prior stroke or thromboembolic event, or known intracardiac thrombus	Bileaflet aortic valve prosthesis and AF	Any mitral valve prosthesis, any caged-ball or tilting-disk aortic-valve prosthesis, multiple mechanical heart valves, or stroke, transient ischemic attack, or cardioembolic event
VTE	VTE >12 mo previously and no other risk factor (eg, provoked and transient)	VTE within previous 3–12 mo, nonsevere thrombophilia, or recurrent VTE	VTE within previous 3 mo, severe thrombophilia, unprovoked VTE, or active cancer (cancer diagnosed ≤6 mo or patient undergoing cancer therapy)

Abbreviations: AF, atrial fibrillation; CHADS2, Congestive heart failure, Hypertension, Age (>65 = 1 point; >75 = 2 points), Diabetes, and Stroke/transient ischemic attack; CHA2DS2-VASc, Congestive heart failure, Hypertension, Age > 75 years, Diabetes, and Stroke/transient ischemic attack, Vascular disease, Age 65-74 years, Sex category; VTE, venous thromboembolism.

Adapted from Douketis JD, Spyropoulos AC, Spencer FA, et al. Perioperative management of antithrombotic therapy: antithrombotic therapy and prevention of thrombosis, 9th ed: American College of Chest Physicians evidence-based clinical practice guidelines. Chest 2012;141(2 Suppl):e330S; with permission.

thrombosis.[46] Another study of 1884 patients (the BRIDGE [Effectiveness of Bridging Anticoagulation for Surgery] trial) with a mean CHADS2 score of 2.3 concluded that foregoing bridging in patients requiring warfarin interruption decreased the risk of bleeding and was noninferior as compared with bridging therapy.[47] However, considerations from the BRIDGE trial cannot be applied universally because oral and maxillofacial surgical patients with a prior history of stroke and those with high CHADS2 scores of 5 to 6 were underrepresented in the studies. Therefore, for patients on warfarin for AF, it seems to be safe to discontinue anticoagulant therapy without any bridging if the CHADS2 score is less than 4 or there is no history of a prior stroke. For patients with a history of recent stroke or CHADS2 scores of 5 to 6, bridging therapy should still be considered.

Warfarin for venous thromboembolism or pulmonary embolism Patients with a history of VTE or PE (provoked from recent surgery, estrogen treatment, pregnancy, lower extremity injury, or air flight time of >8 hours) should be considered candidates for anticoagulation with warfarin for 3 months. Patients with an unprovoked or recurrent VTE (unless confined to the distal veins) or PE are candidates for long-term (indefinite) anticoagulation treatment.[8] Those with a history of provoked VTE/PE and considered high risk for recurrence are patients with active thrombophilic conditions (antithrombin III deficiency, antiphospholipid antibody syndrome, or active cancer) and such individuals are considered good candidates for long-term anticoagulation therapy.

An important factor in the decision to stop warfarin anticoagulation for 5 days versus bridging with LMWH is the time elapsed since a patient's

Table 4
CHADS2 and CHA2DS2-VASc risk stratification scores for subjects with nonvalvular atrial fibrillation

	CHADS2 Score	CHA2DS2-VASc Score
C- Congestive heart failure	1	1
H- Hypertension	1	1
A- Age ≥75 y	1	2
D- Diabetes	1	1
S- Stroke/TIA	2	2
V- Vascular disease (prior MI, PAD, or aortic plaque)	—	1
A- Age 65–74 y	—	1
S- Sex category (female sex)	—	1
Maximum score	6	9

Abbreviations: CHADS2, Congestive heart failure, Hypertension, Age (>65 = 1 point; >75 = 2 points), Diabetes, and Stroke/transient ischemic attack; CHA2DS2-VASc, Congestive heart failure, Hypertension, Age > 75 years, Diabetes, and Stroke/transient ischemic attack, Vascular disease, Age 65-74 years, Sex category; MI, myocardial infarction; PAD, peripheral artery disease; TIA, transient ischemic attack.
From Gage BF, Waterman AD, Shannon W, et al. Validation of clinical classification schemes for predicting stroke: results from the National Registry of Atrial Fibrillation. JAMA 2001;285(22):2867; with permission.

last incident of VTE/PE. In patients with a very recent thrombotic event (within 3 months), invasive elective surgery should be postponed until the appropriate duration of anticoagulation has been achieved. For those with a recent DVT/PE (within 3 months) requiring invasive surgery that cannot be postponed, bridging should be used, secondary to a risk of 50% thrombosis recurrence in the absence of anticoagulation.[2,3,5] In patients at low risk of recurrence (DVT/PE >12 months) and no additional prothrombotic risk factors, warfarin can be stopped for 5 days without bridging. For individuals at moderate thromboembolic risk (history of DVT/PE between 3 and 12 months before elective invasive surgery, active thrombophilia, or cancer), concern for incidence of thrombosis needs to be balanced against the perioperative risks of bleeding in the event of bridging. This patient population can either forgo bridging or receive prophylactic dosing with LMWH when the intraoperative or postoperative risk of bleeding is considered high.[2,27,40,45]

Warfarin for mechanical heart valves There is a high risk of major embolic events (4 per 100 patient-years) for patients with mechanical cardiac valves in the absence of anticoagulation.[48] However, embolism risks can be decreased (1 per 100 patient-years) when prescribing warfarin therapy after prosthetic valve replacement surgery and the risk is estimated to be twice as high for those with mitral mechanical heart valves as compared with aortic valves.[48] Patients with bileaflet aortic valve prosthesis in the absence of a history of stroke or cardioembolic event are considered low risk and could stop warfarin 5 days preoperatively.[3] Individuals with bileaflet mechanical aortic valves in the presence of AF are considered a moderate risk. Patients considered to be at high risk of thromboembolism in the absence of anticoagulation according to the 2012 ACCP guidelines include those with mechanical valves in the mitral position, older aortic valves (ball-cage, tilting-disk), multiple mechanical heart valves, and a history of cerebrovascular of cardioembolic events.[3] Therefore, it is suggested that patients in the high- and moderate-risk categories be considered for bridging therapy.[2,9]

Step 4: bridging therapy considerations
Patients at high risk for thromboembolism should be considered for bridging therapy, but perioperative bleeding risks need to be weighed against antithrombotic benefit when considering such treatment. Several trials have described increased bleeding risks (including major bleeding events) in those prescribed bridging interventions with no significant benefit regarding thromboembolic effects.[46,47,49] Therefore, until more evidence becomes available, bridging with therapeutic doses of parenteral anticoagulants should be considered only in cases of high-risk of thrombosis such as:

- Patients with AF and a history of recent stroke or CHADS2 score of 5 to 6,
- Those with recent VTE/PE (within 3 months),
- Individuals with mechanical mitral valves, and
- Patients with older and bileaflet aortic valves along with a history of stroke or other cardio-embolic event.[2]

Bridging can be accomplished with therapeutic doses of either LMWH or UFH (LMWH used more often than UFH) in the high-risk case examples presented and either LMWH or UFH recommended when bridging is considered for AF and VTE[50] (**Table 5**). In Europe, only UFH is approved for patients that have received mechanical heart valves secondary to lack of investigation assessing efficacy of LMWH in this setting.[51] In contrast, the 2014 American College

Table 5
Bridging regimens

Anticoagulant	Therapeutic Dose	Prophylactic Dose
Enoxaparin	1 mg/kg SC BID or 1.5 mg/kg SC QD	30 mg SC BID or 40 mg SC QD
Dalteparin	120 U/kg SC BID or 200 U/kg SC QD	5000 U SC QD
Unfractionated heparin	Dose needed to achieve an aPTT 1.5–2 times the control aPTT	5000–7500 U SC BID

Abbreviations: aPTT, activated thromboplastin time; BID, twice a day; QD, daily; SC, subcutaneous.

of Cardiology/American Heart Association Guideline for Management of Patients with Valvular Heart Disease and 2012 ACCP Guidelines on the Perioperative Management of Antithrombotic Therapy recommends that either UFH and LMWH can be used in patients with mechanical valves.[3,9] In patients prescribed warfarin for VTE of PE that occurred less than 3 months before planned invasive surgical procedure and not categorized as high risk for thromboembolism, prophylactic doses of LMWH or UFH can be used as bridging therapy. Such an approach would reduce thromboembolic risk as well as that of perioperative bleeding compared with a therapeutic dose bridging model.[3]

Bridging with LMWH or UFH can be started 24 to 48 hours after warfarin cessation (3 days before the planned procedure) to allow INR values to drift toward the normal range. Because UFH has a shorter half-life, an UFH infusion needs to be discontinued 4 to 6 hours before the procedure, but when LMWH is used for bridging, the last dose should be administered at one-half the daily dose and delivered 24 hours before the planned oral/maxillofacial operation.[31]

Restarting warfarin therapy Warfarin is usually restarted within 12 to 24 hours after the procedure provided adequate hemostasis has been established. When prior bridging treatment was deemed necessary, LMWH can be restarted 24 hours after surgery for procedures within the low bleeding risk category (HAS BLED score <3) and 48 to 72 hours after surgery for those with high bleeding risk (HAS BLED score >3). Bridging therapy can then be discontinued when the INR has been increased into the desired therapeutic range within 48 hours.[45]

Perioperative Management of Patients on Fondaparinux

Preoperative treatment with anticoagulants can expose patients undergoing surgery to higher risks of perioperative bleeding. However, there are limited data available for perioperative management of those taking fondaparinux. Effects of this medication can last 3 to 5 half-lives or 3 to 4 days. Patients taking fondaparinux should discontinue it 72 to 96 hours before elective invasive surgery when treated with therapeutic doses (7.5 mg SC) and for 24 hours for those receiving prophylactic doses (eg, 2.5 mg SC). The only data currently available is for perioperative management of fondaparinux for those scheduled for coronary artery bypass surgery and the findings support discontinuation of this medication 36 hours before surgery.[52]

Perioperative Management of Patients on New Oral Anticoagulants

Relatively short half-lives of this class of medications permit discontinuation of these agents closer to the day of scheduled invasive oral and maxillofacial surgery. In addition, bridging therapy is not typically needed, because thrombotic risks are not increased significantly with NOAC medication interruption in addition to concerns that bridging can also increase periprocedural bleeding.[7,53] There are some data available showing that certain procedures can be performed without stopping warfarin and can also be performed while continuing NOACs. Evidence from a registry involving 2179 patients taking NOACs undergoing superficial skin surgeries, dental extractions, cataract surgery, and endoscopic procedures detected only rare bleeding events (0.5%).[54] There are also data that certain cosmetic/dermatologic procedures can be performed safely on those taking NOACs or interventions performed with patients on dabigatran that did not result in excessive bleeding.[55] However, until more studies become available to assess the safety of continuing NOACs perioperatively in the oral and maxillofacial patient population, it may be more prudent to stop such medications for procedures, except those with minimal risk of bleeding (dental cleaning and fillings or minor skin procedures).[56]

Guidelines exist for perioperative management of patients taking NOACs and these recommendations are summarized in **Table 6**[57,58] with considerations being based on individual patient renal

Table 6
Recommendations for NOAC discontinuation before elective surgery

Guideline	Cr Cl (mL/min)	Dabigatran		Rivaroxaban		Apixaban		Edoxaban	
		High-Risk Bleeding	Low-Risk Bleeding	High-Risk Bleeding	Low-Risk Bleeding	High-Risk Bleeding	Low-Risk Bleeding	High-Risk Bleeding	Low-Risk Bleeding
European Heart Rhythm Association	≥80	≥48 h	≥24 h	≥48 h	≥24 h	≥48 h	≥24 h	Not addressed	
	50–80	≥72 h	≥36 h	≥48 h	≥24 h	≥48 h	≥24 h		
	30–50	≥96 h	≥48 h	≥48 h	≥24 h	≥48 h	≥24 h		
	15–30	Not indicated	Not indicated	≥48 h	≥36 h	≥48 h	≥36 h		
Australasian Society of Thrombosis and Hemostasis	≥50	≥72 h	≥48 h	≥72 h	≥24 h	≥72 h	≥24 h	Not addressed	
	30–49	≥96–120 h	≥72 h	≥72 h	≥24 h	≥96 h	≥72 h		
Working Group on perioperative Haemostasis and the French Study Group on Thrombosis and Haemostasis	Not addressed	≥5 d	≥24 h	≥5 d	≥24 h	≥5 d	≥24 h	Not addressed	
Manufacturer recommendations	≥50	≥24–48 h		≥24 h (Cr Cl and bleeding risk not addressed)		≥48 h (Cr Cl not addressed)	≥24 h	≥24 h (Cr Cl and bleeding risk not addressed)	
	<50	≥72–120 h							

Abbreviations: Cr Cl, creatine clearance; NOAC, newer oral anticoagulants.

function and relation to potential bleeding risks. Within these guidelines, bleeding risk has been defined differently according to surgeries with a high 2-day postoperative hemorrhagic risk (or procedures lasting >45 min) of 2% to 4% in contrast to procedures considered low bleeding risk interventions (0%–2% 2-d risk of major bleeding).[37]

Perioperative Oral Anticoagulants and Emergency Surgery

Patients prescribed anticoagulants and presenting for emergency or trauma surgery should discontinue antithrombotic medications and institute supportive measures protecting against hemorrhagic risks. Warfarin anticoagulation can be assessed by following INR levels, but effects from NOAC medications cannot always be quantified with coagulation testing. An increased prothrombin time is expected in patients on rivaroxaban, but prothrombin time is insensitive for those taking apixaban. A prolonged aPTT occurs in the presence of dabigatran; however, the INR/prothrombin time/aPTT values do not correlate with the amount of NOAC medication found in plasma. These tests serve merely as a confirmation of the presence of such agents in the patient's circulation.

Warfarin therapy can be reversed by administration of fresh frozen plasma (10–15 mL/kg) in addition to a slow infusion of vitamin K (5–10 mg) in urgent and emergent cases. The prothrombin complex concentrate can be superior to fresh frozen plasma in reversing vitamin K antagonists because of the (1) rapid speed of infusion, (2) lack of need for crossmatching, (3) small volume to be infused, and (4) effectiveness of reversal (however, higher incidence of thromboembolism). A 4-factor prothrombin complex concentrate (K Centra-containing factors II, VII, IX, and X) is currently approved by the US Food and Drug Administration for reversal of warfarin.[22]

Continuous risk assessment regarding timing or urgency of a surgical procedure is warranted in patients prescribed with NOAC agents because a 24- to 48-hour hold of such medications can result in a normal coagulation status. Elimination of anticoagulation effects from dabigatran with hemodialysis can be considered for urgent and emergent surgeries in patients taking this medication. In addition, idarucizumab (Praxbind; administered in 2 consecutive infusions or boluses of 2.5 g each) has recently been approved by the US Food and Drug Administration for reversal of dabigatran, and currently reserved for patients requiring truly emergent surgery. Idarucizumab is an antibody fragment that attaches to the thrombin binding

site of dabigatran, leading to complete reversal of anticoagulation effects within minutes.[59] Andexanet alfa, a modified recombinant factor Xa, is being investigated for reversal of all anti–Xa inhibitors (both oral and intravenous), with evidence of effects within minutes of administration.[60] Aripazine (ciraparantag, PER-977) is a small molecule that interacts with the anticoagulant agents through noncovalent hydrogen bonding and electrostatic interactions. Aripazine is now in phase II clinical trials and seems to inhibit nearly all anticoagulants with the exception of vitamin K antagonists and argatroban.[61] In dire emergency situations, off-label administration of prothrombin complex concentrate and recombinant factor VII can be used during life-threatening bleeding scenarios.[22,61]

PERIPROCEDURAL MANAGEMENT OF PATIENTS ON COAGULATION-ALTERING THERAPY

The concern with any anticoagulated patient during routine dental and minimally invasive procedures is the location of occurrence and how to best manage those with the development of a hematoma.[62] A significant hematoma complication could result in patient airway compromise or disruption of surgical/interventional repair, require an additional intervention to evacuate the clot, compromise granulation ability, adversely affect any suture closures, or result in potential of neurologic injury/damage[4] because certain peripheral procedures or soft tissue injections in anticoagulated patients could result in hematoma formation where manual vessel compression could be difficult or not possible. These situations represent several potential adverse events and compromising hematoma formation that can result in neurologic dysfunction from mechanical compression.[13,63]

The scope of interventional procedures in oral and maxillofacial health care can be multifaceted (including nerve blocks, joint injections, cancer pain interventions, soft tissue procedures, trigger point injections, etc). Bleeding complications from these techniques can include hematoma formation, hemarthroses, and SC ecchymosis. The dental literature has issued guidelines for management of patients taking antiplatelet, anticoagulant, and antifibrinolytic medications and subsequently planning interventional procedures.[64–67] A strong body of information, indirectly related to the oral and maxillofacial surgery patient, can also be gained from the American Society of Regional Anesthesia and Pain Medicine.[2,4,68] Many of these published recommendations for high- and moderate-risk procedures are similar; however, distinctions do exist and the more recent publications indicates that during low-risk procedures that less stringent criteria could be acceptable.[2,69] Regardless of published guidelines consulted, it remains important to follow a formal risk assessment with decisions performed in conjunction with the treating physicians management of a patient's anticoagulant therapy when necessary.[63]

Periprocedural Management of Patients on Unfractionated Heparin

Before performing interventional procedures, clinicians should review a patient's medical history to determine if concurrent medications or evidence of organ dysfunction could alter responses to heparin therapy (metabolism, excretion) or increase bleeding risk.[67] Guidelines exist that recommend for patients receiving heparin 4 days or longer to have a platelet count measured.[4,70] For patients receiving 5000 U of SC UFH twice daily for DVT

prophylaxis, there are no contraindications to interventional procedures and no delay is necessary between performing the procedure and administration of subsequent SC UFH.[4,67,71] In those receiving SC heparin greater than 10,000 U daily or more than twice daily heparin dosing, safety data to make formal recommendations in all planned interventional procedures are not available. There are reports that three times daily heparin dosing can increase bleeding risks, however, such a practice is maintained in patients on thrice daily heparin at many facilities.[68,71,72] In patients receiving IV UFH, infusions should be stopped 2 to 6 hours with documentation of a normal aPTT before any seriously invasive oral and maxillofacial procedure is undertaken[4] (**Table 7**).

Considerations for invasive interventional procedures
When performing certain interventional procedures, consider a 4-hour interval after discontinuing heparin therapy and conducting such techniques,

Table 7
Periprocedural management of antithrombotics

Drug	Data Adapted from the 2015 Interventional Pain ASRA Guidelines		
	When to Discontinue		
	High and Intermediate Risk	Low Risk	When to Restart
Intravenous heparin	4 h	4 h	2 h
SC heparin	8–10 h	8–10 h	2 h
LMWH: Prophylactic dosing (enoxaparin 30 mg SC BID enoxaparin 40 mg SC QD deltaparin 5000 U SC QD)	12 h	12 h	4 h after a low risk procedure; 12–24 h after a intermediate or high risk procedure
LMWH: *Therapeutic dosing* (enoxaparin1.5 mg/kg SC QD or 1 mg/kg SC BID dalteparin 120 U SC BID or 200 U QD)	24 h	24 h	4 h after a low risk procedure; 12–24 h after a intermediate or high risk procedure
Warfarin	5 d and normal INR	Discontinuation may not be necessary if INR <3	24 h
Fondaparinux 2.5 mg SC QD	4 d	Shared assessment and risk stratification, a 2 half-life interval discontinuation may be considered	24 h
Dabigatran	4–5 d (normal renal function) 6 d (impaired renal function)		24 h
Rivaroxaban	3 d		24 h
Apixaban	3–5 d		24 h

Abbreviations: ASRA, American Society of Regional Anesthesia and Pain Medicine; BID, twice daily; INR, international normalized ratio; LMWH, low molecular weight heparin; QD, once daily; SC, subcutaneous.

especially for high-risk procedures. In addition, there are some guidelines that suggest waiting 2 hours after interventional procedures before restarting heparin and evidence of traumatic interventional procedures may requires a 24-hour interval before resuming intravenous heparin.[2] It is recommended that, when possible, interventional techniques occur 8 to 10 hours after last the SC heparin used for DVT prophylaxis and heparin restarted 2 hours after performing such procedures.[2] Bleeding risks associated with three times daily heparin are unknown and it is preferred that interventional techniques be conducted on those receiving twice daily heparin until more definitive data are available.[2]

Periprocedural Management of Patients on Low-Molecular-Weight Heparin

When performing invasive interventions, considerations for delay of 12 hours in patients receiving prophylactic dosing of SC LMHW (either enoxaparin 40 mg SC daily or 30 mg twice daily) should be considered.[4,5,27] In those that receive therapeutic LMWH (enoxaparin 1 mg/kg SC twice daily or 1.5 mg/kg daily and dalteparin 120 U/kg twice daily or 200 U/kg daily), an even longer delay (24 hours) after the last LMWH injection is recommended by the 2010 ASRA guidelines.[4] Postprocedurally, once daily LMWH for prophylaxis can be administered 6 to 8 hours later after confirmation of normal hemostasis. A second postprocedural LMWH prophylaxis dose could occur 24 hours later[4] (see **Table 7**).

Periprocedural Management of Patients on Warfarin

As mentioned, anticoagulation with warfarin therapy should be stopped 4 to 5 days before any planned invasive interventional procedures along with documentation of INR within the normal reference range on the day of the invasive procedure.[73] The 2010 ASRA guidelines suggest that in those receiving preoperative warfarin (typically the night before) that an INR be checked if the first dose was given greater than 24 hours before or if a second warfarin dose was administered.[4] In addition, concurrent medications affecting hemostatic mechanisms such as antiplatelet agents (aspirin, nonsteroidal antiinflammatory drugs, etc) can increase hematoma formation and should be investigated.[4,74]

An INR of less than 1.5 correlates well with clotting factor levels of at least 40%. With an INR between 1.5 and 3, caution should be exercised along with a review of patient medical records to determine if other agents affecting hemostasis (medications not effecting INR) are present. In such a situation as combined anticoagulation therapy, close observation/evaluation should occur in the periprocedural period. For those with an INR of greater than 3, warfarin should be held or reduced before performance of invasive intervention(s) were hematoma development could prove detrimental to procedure outcome.[4,27,66]

When performing high- or intermediate-risk techniques or interventions, consideration for holding warfarin therapy could be necessary (a period of 5 days and normal INR documented); however, during low-risk interventional procedures, there is evidence that it is safe to proceed despite a therapeutic INR, as long as it is less than 3.0 and no serious deleterious or unsafe effects are possible should hematoma development occur.[69,75] It is further recommended that such a decision involve a shared risk assessment, stratification, and management decision in conjunction with the prescribing physician.[2,68]

Periprocedural Management of Patients on Fondaparinux

The true risks of hematoma formation in those receiving fondaparinux remains unknown and many subsequent clinical studies evaluating such risks were performed with stringent criteria that may not always be feasible in all routine clinical situations. Therefore, if fondaparinux is being administered, then the 2010 ASRA guidelines for performing interventions where hematoma formation could result in patient morbidity recommends that these techniques should only occur under stringent criteria and if these criteria cannot be met, other thromboprophylaxis therapy should be considered. In addition, these considerations apply only to patients treated with prophylactic doses of fondaparinux (2.5 mg SC daily) and invasive interventions or surgery should probably not be performed for those on therapeutic doses of fondaparinux (5–10 mg SC daily) given the increased risk of compromising hematoma formation.[27,68]

For patients taking fondaparinux and scheduled for low-risk interventional procedures, 2 half-life intervals should be adequate before performing such techniques. In more moderate- or high-risk interventional procedures, considerations for 5 half-lives or a 3- to 4-day discontinuation interval for fondaparinux is recommended before the intervention. Fondaparinux can be resumed 24 hours after the procedure.[2,27,69]

Periprocedural Management of Patients on New Oral Anticoagulants

An important consideration is awareness of the half-life of any particular agent to determine amount of time (numbers of days) in which the medication should be discontinued before performing interventional procedures. Another important consideration for all patients prescribed oral anticoagulation therapy is to recommend against the concurrent use of medications that affect other components of the clotting mechanisms.

When performing low-risk interventional procedures, a 2 half-life discontinuation interval could be considered for those taking the NOACs, a shared risk decision that should be made in conjunction with the prescribing physicians. When performing moderate and high-risk interventional procedures in patients prescribed NOACs (dabigatran, rivaroxaban, or apixaban), a 5 half-life period of discontinuation of the agent is recommended. For dabigatran, this corresponds to a 4- to 5-day discontinuation period except for those patients with renal dysfunction (end-stage renal disease) where a 6-day delay is recommended because renal compromise can increase the half-life from 8 to 14 hours to 28 hours. Patients on rivaroxaban should have the medication discontinued for 3 days and apixaban 3 to 5 days before intermediate- and high-risk interventional procedures.[2,69,70]

SUMMARY

Coagulation-altering therapy should be based on patient-specific condition (renal, hepatic, cardiac) and surgery-related (elective, degree of invasiveness, trauma, cancer) issues to effectively proceed with surgery and/or perform interventional procedures. The potential for confusion can exist from the significant number of prophylactic and therapeutic coagulation-altering medications that patients have been prescribed. Therefore, understanding its complexity is essential and decisions about performing surgery and interventional techniques in patients receiving such therapy need to be made on an individual basis depending on a host of factors, including (1) merely identifying risks and following consensus guidelines will not completely eliminate hematoma formation, complications from thrombus, or risks of serious bleeding, (2) considering selection of alternative techniques or delay procedures for the suggested period(s) of time for patients with unacceptable risks, (3) manufacturer-suggested anticoagulant medication dosing guidelines should be followed, (4) appropriate optimization of coagulation status and timing of surgery, proper selection of bridging needs and options, and remain cognizant of appropriate anticoagulation level monitoring, and (5) extending consideration of appropriate dosing/timing intervals during perioperative and periprocedural interventions.

REFERENCES

1. Bracey AW. Perioperative management of antithrombotic and antiplatelet therapy. Tex Heart Inst J 2015; 42:239–42.
2. Narouze S, Benzon HT, Provenzano DA, et al. Interventional spine and pain procedures in patients on antiplatelet and anticoagulant medications: guidelines from the American Society of Regional Anesthesia and Pain Medicine, the European Society of Regional Anaesthesia and Pain Therapy, the American Academy of Pain Medicine, the International Neuromodulation Society, the North American Neuromodulation Society, and the World Institute of Pain. Reg Anesth Pain Med 2015;40:182–212.
3. Douketis JD, Spyropoulos AC, Spencer FA, et al. Perioperative management of antithrombotic therapy: antithrombotic therapy and prevention of thrombosis, 9th ed: American College of Chest Physicians Evidence-Based Clinical Practice Guidelines. Chest 2012;141:e326S–50S.
4. Horlocker TT, Wedel DJ, Rowlingson JC, et al. Regional anesthesia in the patient receiving antithrombotic or thrombolytic therapy: American Society of Regional Anesthesia and Pain Medicine evidence-based guidelines (third edition). Reg Anesth Pain Med 2010;35:64–101.
5. Eisele R, Melzer N, Bramlage P. Perioperative management of anticoagulation. Chirurgie 2014;85: 513–9 [in German].
6. Costa FW, Rodrigues RR, Sousa LH, et al. Local hemostatic measures in anticoagulated patients undergoing oral surgery: a systematized literature review. Acta Cir Bras 2013;28(1):78–83.
7. Madrid C, Sanz M. What influence do anticoagulants have on oral implant therapy? A systematic review. Clin Oral Implants Res 2009;20(Suppl 4):96–106.
8. Kearon C, Akl EA, Comerota AJ, et al. Antithrombotic therapy for VTE disease: antithrombotic therapy and prevention of thrombosis, 9th ed: American College of Chest Physicians evidence-based clinical practice guidelines. Chest 2012;141: e419S–94S.
9. Nishimura RA, Otto CM, Bonow RO, et al. 2014 AHA/ACC guideline for the management of patients with valvular heart disease: a report of the American College of Cardiology/American Heart Association Task Force on practice guidelines. J Am Coll Cardiol 2014;63:e57–185.
10. Pototski M, Amenábar JM. Dental management of patients receiving anticoagulation or antiplatelet treatment. J Oral Sci 2007;49(4):253–8.
11. Cappelleri JC, Fiore LD, Brophy MT, et al. Efficacy and safety of combined anticoagulant and antiplatelet therapy versus anticoagulant monotherapy after mechanical heart-valve replacement: a metaanalysis. Am Heart J 1995;130(3 Pt 1):547–52.

12. Johnson SG, Rogers K, Delate T, et al. Outcomes associated with combined antiplatelet and anticoagulant therapy. Chest 2008;133(4):948–54.

13. Horlocker TT. Regional anaesthesia in the patient receiving antithrombotic and antiplatelet therapy. Br J Anaesth 2011;107(Suppl 1):i96–106.

14. Eriksson BI, Quinlan DJ, Weitz JI. Comparative pharmacodynamics and pharmacokinetics of oral direct thrombin and factor Xa inhibitors in development. Clin Pharmacokinet 2009;48(1):1–22.

15. Greinacher A, Lubenow N. Recombinant hirudin in clinical practice: focus on lepirudin. Circulation 2001;103(10):1479–84.

16. Linnemann B, Greinacher A, Lindhoff-Last E. Alteration of pharmacokinetics of lepirudin caused by anti-lepirudin antibodies occurring after long-term subcutaneous treatment in a patient with recurrent VTE due to Behcets disease. Vasa 2010;39(1):103–7.

17. Rosenquist RW, Brown DL. Neuraxial bleeding: fibrinolytics/thrombolytics. Reg Anesth Pain Med 1998; 23(6 Suppl 2):152–6.

18. Greinacher A. Clinical practice. Heparin-induced thrombocytopenia. N Engl J Med 2015;373:252–61.

19. Tapson VF, Shirvanian S. Venous thromboembolism: identifying patients at risk and establishing prophylaxis. Curr Med Res Opin 2015;31(12):2297–311.

20. Hirsh J, Levine MN. Low molecular weight heparin. Blood 1992;79:1–17.

21. Egan G, Ensom MH. Measuring anti-factor Xa activity to monitor low-molecular-weight heparin in obesity: a critical review. Can J Hosp Pharm 2015; 68:33–47.

22. Daniels PR. Peri-procedural management of patients taking oral anticoagulants. BMJ 2015;351: h2391.

23. Levy JH, Faraoni D, Spring JL, et al. Managing new oral anticoagulants in the perioperative and intensive care unit setting. Anesthesiology 2013;118: 1466–74.

24. Mandernach MW, Beyth RJ, Rajasekhar A. Apixaban for the prophylaxis and treatment of deep vein thrombosis and pulmonary embolism: an evidence-based review. Ther Clin Risk Manag 2015;11: 1273–82.

25. Minor C, Tellor KB, Armbruster AL. Edoxaban, a novel oral factor Xa inhibitor. Ann Pharmacother 2015;49:843–50.

26. Tafur AJ, McBane R, Wysokinski WE, et al. Predictors of major bleeding in peri-procedural anticoagulation management. J Thromb Haemost 2012;10: 261–7.

27. Wahl MJ, Pinto A, Kilham J, et al. Dental surgery in anticoagulated patients–stop the interruption. Oral Surg Oral Med Oral Pathol Oral Radiol 2015; 119(2):136–57.

28. Roldán V, Marín F, Manzano-Fernández S, et al. The HAS-BLED score has better prediction accuracy for major bleeding than CHADS2 or CHA2DS2-VASc scores in anticoagulated patients with atrial fibrillation. J Am Coll Cardiol 2013;62:2199–204.

29. Apostolakis S, Lane DA, Buller H, et al. Comparison of the CHADS2, CHA2DS2-VASc and HAS-BLED scores for the prediction of clinically relevant bleeding in anticoagulated patients with atrial fibrillation: the AMADEUS trial. Thromb Haemost 2013; 110;1074–9.

30. Omran H, Bauersachs R, Rübenacker S, et al. The HAS-BLED score predicts bleedings during bridging of chronic oral anticoagulation. Results from the national multicentre BNK Online bRiDging REgistRy (BORDER). Thromb Haemost 2012;108: 65–73.

31. Baron TH, Kamath PS, McBane RD. Management of antithrombotic therapy in patients undergoing invasive procedures. N Engl J Med 2013;368:2113–24.

32. Ferrieri GB, Castiglioni S, Carmagnola D, et al. Oral surgery in patients on anticoagulant treatment without therapy interruption. J Oral Maxillofac Surg 2007;65(6):1149–54.

33. Palamaras I, Semkova K. Perioperative management of and recommendations for antithrombotic medications in dermatological surgery. Br J Dermatol 2015;172:597–605.

34. Perry DJ, Noakes TJ, Helliwell PS, et al. Guidelines for the management of patients on oral anticoagulants requiring dental surgery. Br Dent J 2007;203: 389–93.

35. Kearon C, Hirsh J. Management of anticoagulation before and after elective surgery. N Engl J Med 1997;336:1506–11.

36. Hylek EM, Regan S, Go AS, et al. Clinical predictors of prolonged delay in return of the international normalized ratio to within the therapeutic range after excessive anticoagulation with warfarin. Ann Intern Med 2001;135:393–400.

37. Spyropoulos AC, Douketis JD. How I treat anticoagulated patients undergoing an elective procedure or surgery. Blood 2012;120:2954–62.

38. Sticherling C, Marin F, Birnie D, et al. Antithrombotic management in patients undergoing electrophysiological procedures: a European Heart Rhythm Association (EHRA) position document endorsed by the ESC Working Group Thrombosis, Heart Rhythm Society (HRS), and Asia Pacific Heart Rhythm Society (APHRS). Europace 2015; 17:1197–214.

39. Amer MZ, Mourad SI, Salem AS, et al. Correlation between International Normalized Ratio values and sufficiency of two different local hemostatic measures in anticoagulated patients. Eur J Dent 2014; 8(4):475–80.

40. Eichhorn W, Burkert J, Vorwig O, et al. Bleeding incidence after oral surgery with continued oral anticoagulation. Clin Oral Investig 2012;16(5):1371–6.

41. Birnie DH, Healey JS, Wells GA, et al. Pacemaker or defibrillator surgery without interruption of anticoagulation. N Engl J Med 2013;368:2084–93.

42. Agarwal S, Hachamovitch R, Menon V. Current trial-associated outcomes with warfarin in prevention of stroke in patients with nonvalvular atrial fibrillation: a meta-analysis. Arch Intern Med 2012;172:623–31 [discussion: 631–3].

43. Kaatz S, Douketis JD, Zhou H, et al. Risk of stroke after surgery in patients with and without chronic atrial fibrillation. J Thromb Haemost 2010;8:884–90.

44. Olesen JB, Torp-Pedersen C, Hansen ML, et al. The value of the CHA2DS2-VASc score for refining stroke risk stratification in patients with atrial fibrillation with a CHADS2 score 0-1: a nationwide cohort study. Thromb Haemost 2012;107:1172–9.

45. Williams LA, Hunter JM, Marques MB, et al. Periprocedural management of patients on anticoagulants. Clin Lab Med 2014;34:595–611.

46. Siegal D, Yudin J, Kaatz S, et al. Periprocedural heparin bridging in patients receiving vitamin K antagonists: systematic review and meta-analysis of bleeding and thromboembolic rates. Circulation 2012;126:1630–9.

47. Douketis JD, Spyropoulos AC, Kaatz S, et al. Perioperative bridging anticoagulation in patients with atrial fibrillation. N Engl J Med 2015;373:823–33.

48. Cannegieter SC, Rosendaal FR, Briët E. Thromboembolic and bleeding complications in patients with mechanical heart valve prostheses. Circulation 1994;89:635–41.

49. Bajkin BV, Popovic SL, Selakovic SD. Randomized, prospective trial comparing bridging therapy using low-molecular-weight heparin with maintenance of oral anticoagulation during extraction of teeth. J Oral Maxillofac Surg 2009;67(5):990–5.

50. Spyropoulos AC, Turpie AG, Dunn AS, et al. Clinical outcomes with unfractionated heparin or low-molecular-weight heparin as bridging therapy in patients on long-term oral anticoagulants: the REGIMEN registry. J Thromb Haemost 2006;4: 1246–52.

51. Hamm CW, Bassand JP, Agewall S, et al. ESC Guidelines for the management of acute coronary syndromes in patients presenting without persistent ST-segment elevation: the task force for the management of acute coronary syndromes (ACS) in patients presenting without persistent ST-segment elevation of the European Society of Cardiology (ESC). Eur Heart J 2011;32:2999–3054.

52. Landenhed M, Johansson M, Erlinge D, et al. Fondaparinux or enoxaparin: a comparative study of postoperative bleeding in coronary artery bypass grafting surgery. Scand Cardiovasc J 2010;44: 100–6.

53. Vanassche T, Lauw MN, Connolly SJ, et al. Heparin bridging in peri-procedural management of new oral anticoagulant: a bridge too far? Eur Heart J 2014;35:1831–3.

54. Beyer-Westendorf J, Gelbricht V, Förster K, et al. Peri-interventional management of novel oral anticoagulants in daily care: results from the prospective Dresden NOAC registry. Eur Heart J 2014;35: 1888–96.

55. Callahan S, Goldsberry A, Kim G, et al. The management of antithrombotic medication in skin surgery. Dermatol Surg 2012;38:1417–26.

56. Ferrandis R, Castillo J, de Andrés J, et al. The perioperative management of new direct oral anticoagulants: a question without answers. Thromb Haemost 2013;110:515–22.

57. Heidbuchel H, Verhamme P, Alings M, et al. Updated European Heart Rhythm Association Practical Guide on the use of non-vitamin K antagonist anticoagulants in patients with non-valvular atrial fibrillation. Europace 2015;17(10):1467–507.

58. Tran H, Joseph J, Young L, et al. New oral anticoagulants: a practical guide on prescription, laboratory testing and peri-procedural/bleeding management. Australasian Society of Thrombosis and Haemostasis. Intern Med J 2014;44:525–36.

59. Pollack CV, Reilly PA, Eikelboom J, et al. Idarucizumab for dabigatran reversal. N Engl J Med 2015; 373:511–20.

60. Siegal DM, Curnutte JT, Connolly SJ, et al. Andexanet alfa for the reversal of factor Xa inhibitor activity. N Engl J Med 2015;373:2413–24.

61. Crowther M, Crowther MA. Antidotes for novel oral anticoagulants: current status and future potential. Arterioscler Thromb Vasc Biol 2015;35:1736–45.

62. Bajkin BV, Urosevic IM, Stankov KM, et al. Dental extractions and risk of bleeding in patients taking single and dual antiplatelet treatment. Br J Oral Maxillofac Surg 2015;53(1):39–43.

63. Mingarro-de-León A, Chaveli-López B, Gavaldá-Esteve C. Dental management of patients receiving anticoagulant and/or antiplatelet treatment. J Clin Exp Dent 2014;6(2):e155–61.

64. Bajkin BV, Vujkov SB, Milekic BR, et al. Risk factors for bleeding after oral surgery in patients who continued using oral anticoagulant therapy. J Am Dent Assoc 2015;146(6):375–81.

65. Bajkin BV, Selaković SD, Mirković SM, et al. Comparison of efficacy of local hemostatic modalities in anticoagulated patients undergoing tooth extractions. Vojnosanit Pregl 2014;71(12):1097–101.

66. Bajkin BV, Bajkin IA, Petrovic BB. The effects of combined oral anticoagulant-aspirin therapy in patients undergoing tooth extractions: a prospective study. J Am Dent Assoc 2012;143(7):771–6.

67. Hong CH, Napeñas JJ, Brennan MT, et al. Frequency of bleeding following invasive dental procedures in patients on low-molecular-weight heparin therapy. J Oral Maxillofac Surg 2010;68(5):975–9.

68. Gogarten W, Vandermeulen E, Van Aken H, et al. Regional anaesthesia and antithrombotic agents: recommendations of the European Society of Anaesthesiology. Eur J Anaesthesiol 2010;27:999–1015.

69. Clemm R, Neukam FW, Rusche B, et al. Management of anticoagulated patients in implant therapy: a clinical comparative study. Clin Oral Implants Res 2015. [Epub ahead of print].

70. Cho YW, Kim E. Is stopping of anticoagulant therapy really required in a minor dental surgery? How about in an endodontic microsurgery? Restor Dent Endod 2013;38(3):113–8.

71. Kämmerer PW, Frerich B, Liese J, et al. Oral surgery during therapy with anticoagulants-a systematic review. Clin Oral Investig 2015;19(2):171–80.

72. King CS, Holley AB, Jackson JL, et al. Twice vs three times daily heparin dosing for thromboembolism prophylaxis in the general medical population: a metaanalysis. Chest 2007;131:507–16.

73. Jimson S, Amaldhas J, Jimson S, et al. Assessment of bleeding during minor oral surgical procedures and extraction in patients on anticoagulant therapy. J Pharm Bioallied Sci 2015;7(Suppl 1):S134–7.

74. Napenas JJ, Hong CH, Brennan MT, et al. The frequency of bleeding complications after invasive dental treatment in patients receiving single and dual antiplatelet therapy. J Am Dent Assoc 2009; 140(6):690–5.

75. Ahmed I, Gertner E. Safety of arthrocentesis and joint injection in patients receiving anticoagulation at therapeutic levels. Am J Med 2012;125:265–9.

Systemic Disease and Bleeding Disorders for the Oral and Maxillofacial Surgeon

Arman G. Haghighi, DDS[a],*,
Rebecca G. Finder, PharmD, BCPS[b], Jeffrey D. Bennett, DMD[c]

KEYWORDS

- Cirrhosis • Kidney disease • Coagulation • Hemostasis • Oral and maxillofacial surgery

KEY POINTS

- There are multiple systemic diseases that have an impact on coagulation of which oral and maxillofacial surgeons must be cognizant.
- Recent evidence has supported the potential for both hypocoagulable and hypercoagulable states in patients with liver and kidney disease with an even less understood impact on prolonged bleeding in the oral cavity.
- These systemic diseases are not limited to diseases affecting the liver, kidney, and bone marrow; however, these diseases are common among the patient population and surgeons must be capable of making appropriate judgment and modifying care appropriately.

Current treatment of patients with systemic diseases, such as liver and kidney disorders, often have the understanding that these patients are inherently at risk for impaired hemostasis and, therefore, altered bleeding. Currently, standard treatments are often based solely on expert opinion and are not evidence based. Recent evidence has supported the potential for both hypocoagulable and hypercoagulable states in patients with liver and kidney disease, with an even less understood impact on prolonged bleeding in the oral cavity. It is, therefore, prudent to understand the impact that these diseases have on patients and the potential effect on hemostasis when choosing treatment options.

LIVER

The liver is a vital player in coagulation and hemostasis. With the production of clotting factors, inhibitors, and proteins involved in the coagulation cascade as well as the ability to clear these products from circulation, hepatic diseases may significantly alter hemostasis. In liver disease processes, decreased production of clotting factors, thrombocytopenia, platelet dysfunction, and increased circulating fibrinolysis activity based on hepatocellular destruction are evident. It is, therefore, judicious to understand some of the more common hepatic disease processes and their role in coagulation.

a Department of Oral and Maxillofacial Surgery, Indiana University, Indianapolis, IN, USA; b Critical Care Pharmacy, Indiana University Health, 1701 N. Senate Blvd, Indianapolis, IN 46202, USA; c Division of Oral and Maxillofacial Surgery, Roudebush VA Medical Center, Indianapolis, IN, USA
* Corresponding author. Department of Oral and Maxillofacial Surgery, 550 University Boulevard, Indianapolis, IN 46202.
E-mail address: armhaghi@iu.edu

Oral Maxillofacial Surg Clin N Am 28 (2016) 461–471
http://dx.doi.org/10.1016/j.coms.2016.06.004
1042-3699/16/$ – see front matter Published by Elsevier Inc.

oralmaxsurgery.theclinics.com

Cirrhosis

Cirrhosis is a chronic condition in which fibrous tissue replaces damaged hepatocytes. This results in a disruption of blood flow through the liver and hepatocellular failure. Blood flow disruption may lead to portal hypertension subsequently causing ascites, peripheral edema, splenomegaly, and varices in the gastrointestinal (GI) tract. Hepatocellular failure also results in decreased albumin and clotting factor synthesis.

The most common classification scheme for determining prognosis and bleeding risk in hepatic disease patients is the Child-Pugh classification with an updated modified Child-Pugh classification now in place. The classification assesses ascites, encephalopathy, bilirubin level, albumin level, and prothrombin time (PT) values as markers with different numeric scores given to each category based on disease progression. These values are added up and ranked as a Child-Pugh class A, B, or C, with class A patients having a better prognosis (estimated 100% 1-year survival) and class C patients having a worse prognosis (predicted 45% 1-year survival). A correlation between Child-Pugh class and increased bleeding time (BT) has not been identified, but it seems likely that higher Child-Pugh score relates to altered coagulopathy.

Another common scoring system used to assess liver disease is the Model for End-Stage Liver Disease (MELD) score, initially used to determine mortality rates in chronic liver disease patients but later found useful in prioritizing candidates for liver transplants rather than using the Child-Pugh score. It is based on a patient's serum bilirubin, creatinine, and international normalized ratio (INR) values to determine survivability. These components are combined into a formula to develop a score that predicts the 3-month mortality in hospitalized patients.

Cirrhosis may be caused by multiple disease processes, including alcoholic liver disease (most common), viral hepatitis, drug induced (eg, acetaminophen toxicity and chronic methotrexate therapy), autoimmune, dysfunction inherited metabolic diseases, and hepatic congestion.

Vitamin K is an essential cofactor in the production of factors II, VII, IX, and X and proteins C, S, and Z, enabling the binding of calcium to these proteins. Diet (green leafy vegetables) is a large source of vitamin K that is absorbed in the small bowel with the aid of bacteria. In some cases of coagulopathy, vitamin K can be used to increase the number of active coagulation factors. This coagulopathy is due to the decreased synthesis of clotting factors (I, II, V, VII, IX, X, XII, and XIII), resulting in increased PT/INR values.

Cirrhosis and Coagulation

Recent studies of coagulation and cirrhotic patients reveal that these patients may not be in a state of hypocoagulation even though bleeding is prolonged by up to 40% of all patients with cirrhosis.[1] Cirrhosis patients may have hypercoagulation or hypocoagulation. This is due to the nondiscrimination in the reduction of both procoagulants and anticoagulants that are synthesized in the liver. These patients typically have elevated levels of von Willebrand factor and factor VIII whereas protein C and antithrombin are reduced. In such cases of hypercoagulation, anticoagulant therapy may be necessary to prevent a hypercoagulable state. Current evidence also suggests that hypercoagulation contributes to hepatic fibrogenesis, where an association of hypercoagulation and increased progression of hepatic fibrosis has been made. It is theorized that microinfarcts from thrombi cause ischemia and hepatic parenchymal death that is eventually replaced with fibrotic tissue.[2,3] Coagulation as a therapeutic option in cirrhotic patients has been largely unexplored and therefore management recommendations have not yet been made.[4]

When measuring coagulation capacity in cirrhotic patients, clinicians often use PT testing in making their assessment. The inherent problem with this test is that it may not be accurate in vivo. PT primarily measures factor VII, the first factor to be depleted during episodes of bleeding (shortest half-life); therefore, the correct assessment of clotting time cannot be obtained through PT because it only primarily depicts a small portion of the coagulation cascade. There is a potential that decreases in coagulation factors and anticoagulation factors balance each other; therefore, PT may be reactive to decreased coagulants but not the decreased anticoagulants. Protein C, for instance, decreases thrombin formation by inhibiting factor V and VIII.[5] A deficiency in protein C makes patients hypercoagulable. It is hypothesized that the ratio of factor VIII to protein C is one of the determinants for hypercoagulability in cirrhotic patients. PT testing should be taken into consideration; however, a more appropriate in vivo test is necessary to obtain a correct depiction of the coagulation status of a patient. Testing, such as thromboelastography (TEG), is becoming increasingly popular in the determination of coagulation status. This is due to TEG's ability to determine platelet function, fibrinolysis, and clot strength. Unfortunately, TEG is only available in a few large institutions and is not readily available.

Platelet counts in cirrhotic patients are also severely affected. Many cirrhotic patients have decreased platelet counts. The theory behind the pathophysiology is that the resultant portal hypertension causes pooling and sequestration of the corpuscle elements of the blood (thrombocyte sequestration in the spleen). New research is under way with the discovery of cytokine thrombopoietin and its effect in cirrhotic patients. Thrombopoietin is largely produced by the liver and results in thrombocyte production in the bone marrow cells.

Multiple methods are available for patients when concerned for a hypocoagulable state. In patients with platelet counts below 50,000/uL, platelet transfusion is commonly initiated prior to surgery, and it has been shown that multiple units of platelets prior to surgery are necessary to make any significant improvement in platelet counts. Desmopressin (DDAVP) has also shown to shorten the BT in cirrhotic patients and can be used as a helpful adjunct for hemostasis in cirrhotic patients.

KIDNEY DISEASE

Systemic disease processes that decrease kidney function have the potential for decreased hemostasis and increased BTs. Some of the more common kidney diseases encountered by an oral and maxillofacial surgeon include acute kidney injury (AKI) and chronic kidney disease (CKD) and, therefore, are the focus of this discussion.

AKI is defined as a rapid decline in renal function and increase in serum creatinine of 50% or 0.5 to 1.0 mg/dL. The risk injury failure loss ESRD (RIFLE) criteria state that patients are at risk for acute kidney injuries when they have a 1.5-fold increase in serum creatinine, a glomerular filtration rate (GFR) decrease of 25%, or urine output less than 0.5 mL/kg/h for 6 hours. Failure is defined as a 2-fold increase in serum creatinine, GFR decrease of 50%, or urine output below 0.5 mL/kg/h for 12 hours. Patients with AKI often gain weight and experience edema due to positive water retention characterized by azotemia. A large portion of acute renal injuries ends with complete resolution.

CKD is defined as kidney damage for over 3 months or a decreased GFR that is below 60 mL/min regardless of cause. Diabetes and hypertension are the most common causes of CKD, with other causes including chronic glomerulonephritis, polycystic kidney disease, obstructive uropathy, and interstitial nephritis. Chronic renal disease is associated with various systemic effects, including hypertention, congestive heart failure, pericarditis, nausea, vomiting, loss of appetite, lethargy, somnolence, confusion, peripheral neuropathy, and uremic seizures.

Kidney Disease and Coagulation

Patients with kidney disease are susceptible to increased bleeding and at times increased thrombi formation. Bleeding disorders are a result of the insufficient function of platelets, the coagulation cascade, and/or activation of the fibrinolysis system. Hypercoagulability is a result of disorders of the coagulation regulatory factors as well as platelet hyperactivity.[6]

In renal-impaired patients, decreased renal function has an increased effect on prescribed anticoagulants due to reduced clearance, thereby increasing hemostasis time. Renal-impaired patients on hemodialysis are also regularly administered anticoagulants, such as heparin, during treatments, resulting in antithrombin III and factor Xa inactivation and reducing hemostasis.

Platelet function is reduced in patients with renal disease. This is due to the altered platelet alpha granules with an increased ATP/ADP ratio, reduced serotonin content, and increased calcium content.[7] Uremic patients platelets demonstrate degranulated arachidonic acid and prostaglandin metabolism with impaired synthesis/release of thromboxane A_2.[7] This leads to reduced adhesions and aggregation of platelets. Uremic patients have also been shown to decrease the amount of glycoprotein (GP) Ib on platelets due to probable high proteolysis, impeding the ability of platelets to bind to vessel walls.[8]

Drug interactions with hemostasis are highly modified in uremic patients. β-Lactam antibiotics and third-generation cephalosporins potentially interfere with ADP receptors and interfere with the function of platelet membranes depending on dose and duration. Aspirin, a commonly used irreversible antiplatelet, has been shown to have an increased effect in uremic patients when compared with patients with normal kidney function, causing increased BTs.[9] Many commonly used anticoagulants are eliminated through the kidney, and these medications can accumulate in uremic patients. Anticoagulants with potential for accumulation include low-molecular-weight heparins, direct factor Xa inhibitors, and direct thrombin inhibitors.

Patients with renal failure also have the potential for thromboembolism[10] with an increased risk of pulmonary embolism[11] and a 2-fold increased risk of thromboembolism.[12] An increased risk of thromboembolism is associated with a GFR below 75 mL/min/1.73 m^2 and can be due to albuminuria.[13] This hypercoagulable potential is multifactorial in etiology. Increased levels of fibrinogen in CKD patients are attributed to proinflammatory markers interleukin-6 and C-reactive protein,[14] elevated plasma tissue factor (TF),[15] and proinflammation transcription factors nuclear factor κB and protease-activated receptor-1.[16] Some studies also show decreased levels of coagulation factors XIIa/VIIa, protein c complex, and thrombin-antithrombin complexes.[17]

Chronic renal insufficiency, like cirrhotic livers, possess the potential for the hypercoagulable state as well as increased difficulty in obtaining hemostasis. When evaluating these patients, other comorbidities of patients that can be contributory as well as medications that patients may be taking should be taken into consideration. Hemodialysis patients with fistulas and centrally placed lines should be considered a higher risk for thrombus formation. Great care should be taken with these patients, and appropriate work-up and testing can aid in a clinician's assessment.

BONE MARROW FAILURE

Multiple causes exist for the loss of hematopoietic bone marrow cells. The most notable etiologies that damage bone marrow cells are malignancy (eg, leukemia) and chemotherapy medications that target these cells. The resultant loss of hematopoietic bone marrow cells possesses the potential to affect hemostasis and increase BTs by having an impact on megakaryocytes, the progenitor cells for platelets.[18] An oral health care provider may be the first to recognize the early stages of bone marrow failure, because oral bleeding that is plaque-free is often the first sign of bone marrow failure or damage.[19]

DISEASES AFFECTING DRUG METABOLISM

Several factors can affect the normal hemostatic balance – long-term drug therapy, vascular volume expansion, surgical blood loss, and preexisting coagulopathies and systemic diseases. Acute or chronic diseases that affect liver and kidney function markedly affect metabolism and excretion of medications. Drug-metabolizing enzymes may be impaired and significantly alter elimination, which could lead to significant adverse drug reactions in patients with liver disease.[20]

Impaired renal function in CKD patients has consequences for medications not only excreted by the kidneys but also cleared nonrenally. Renal impairment leads to changes in absorption, plasma protein binding, drug transport, and/or tissue distribution and may even affect hepatic and GI metabolism. Uremic toxins accumulated in CKD and end-stage renal disease (ESRD) cause down-regulation of drug-metabolizing enzymes (CYP3A4/F, CYP2C9, CYP2D6, and CYP2C19)

and transporters. It is, therefore, important to assess hepatic and renal function when prescribing most medications.[20]

New Oral Anticoagulants

Consideration of the new oral anticoagulants (dabigatran, rivaroxaban, edoxaban, and apixaban) and their effects on hemostasis in patients with hepatic or renal dysfunction is essential. The new oral anticoagulants and their alterations due to renal and hepatic dysfunction are briefly reviewed. Recommendations for dosing, discontinuation, and reversal of oral anticoagulants and antiplatelets are found in **Table 1**.[21–35]

Dabigatran (Pradaxa®) is a direct factor II inhibitor, with its impact on coagulation assays at recommended therapeutic doses, and displays an increase in median peak activated partial thromboplastin time (aPTT) by 2 times control, with relatively no elevation in INR.[36] Dabigatran must be renally adjusted because 80% of the medication undergoes renal elimination. Therefore, it is not an optimal choice in patients with ESRD or a creatinine clearance less than 15 mL/min.[36] Dabigatran, in comparison to warfarin, has a lower bleeding risk, including intracranial, in patients less than 75 years of age; however, the incidence of GI bleeding is higher. Although no dosing recommendation exists in patients with hepatic impairment, the mechanism of action of dabigatran, as a prodrug needing in vivo hepatic conversion to its active form, warrants additional thought.[36,37] The effect of dabigatran on dental treatment includes bleeding caused by specific, reversible prevention of thrombin-mediated effects and inhibition of platelet aggregation. Hemorrhage may occur depending on multiple variables, including intensity of anticoagulation and patient susceptibility; therefore, medical consult is suggested.

The commonly used oral anti-Xa inhibitors (rivaroxaban, apixaban, and edoxaban) were designed to have predictable pharmacokinetics negating the need for routine laboratory monitoring. Coagulation assays, such as PT/INR, aPTT, and anti-Xa activity, are variably affected by these new oral anticoagulants. Edoxaban (Savaysa), rivaroxaban (Xarelto), and apixaban (Eliquis) have approximately 50%, 33%, and 25% renal elimination, respectively; therefore, it is recommended to avoid the use of these agents in CKD stage 4 and stage 5 patients.[37–40] Use of the oral anti-Xa inhibitors is not recommended in patients with hepatic dysfunction equal to a Child-Pugh class B or C.[38–40] There are circumstances in which monitoring of anticoagulant effect may be indicated,

Table 1
Common anticoagulants and antiplatelets adjustments in the hepatic and renal impaired

Characteristic	Dabigatran (Pradaxa®)[21]	Warfarin (Coumadin®)[22]	Aspirin[23]	Rivaroxaban (Xarelto®)[24]	Apixiban (Eliquis®)[25]	Edoxaban (Savaysa®)[26]	Clopidogrel (Plavix®)[27]	Prasugrel (Effient®)[28]	Ticagrelor (Brilinta®)[29,30]
Mechanism of action	Direct thrombin (factor II) inhibitor	Vitamin K antagonist; inhibits factors II, VII, IX, X and proteins C and S	Antithrombin III activator	Direct factor Xa inhibitor			Inhibits P2Y$_{12}$ of ADP receptors		
Approach for hepatic dysfunction	No dosage adjustment; prodrug	No dosage adjustment; monitor INR closely in obstructive jaundice, hepatitis, and cirrhosis	Avoid use in severe liver disease	Avoid in moderate or severe impairment	Avoid in severe impairment	Mild impairment no dosage adjustment; avoid in moderate to severe impairment	Caution; prolonged platelet aggregation and mean BT with severe impairment	No dosage adjustment	Avoid in severe impairment
Approach for renal dysfunction[31]	No dosage adjustment unless CrCl <50 mL/min and on concomitant P-gp inhibitor	No dosage adjustment; increased risk of bleeding	Avoid use if CrCl <10 mL/min	Renal adjustment required	Renal adjustment required; avoid if CrCl <25 mL/min	Dose reduction if CrCl 15–50 mL/min Avoid if CrCl >95 mL/min or <15 mL/min	No dosage adjustment		
Reversal agents[32–35]	Idarucizumab (Praxbind)	Vitamin K, FFP, PCC	Platelet transfusion; DDAVP	Andexanet alfa (Andexanet); PCC			Platelet transfusion; DDAVP		Aminocaproic acid, tranexamic acid

Abbreviations: ADP, adenosine diphosphate; CrCl, creatinine clearance; DDAVP, desmopressin; FFP, fresh frozen plasma; PCC, prothombin complex concentrate; P-gp, P-glycoprotein.
Data from Refs.[21–35]

such as treatment failure, bleeding, renal or hepatic dysfunction, and perioperative monitoring. The clinical relevance of these agents' serum levels warrants further study.

Antibiotics

Rare reports suggest certain antibiotics may potentiate bleeding. The most common culprits are the second-generation and third-generation cephalosporins and antifungal drugs.[41] Hypothesized mechanisms for antibiotic-induced coagulopathy consist of myelosuppression, immune-mediated destruction of thrombocytes and coagulation factors; suppression of vitamin K epoxide reductase may inhibit biosynthesis of factors II, VII, IX, and X. It is unclear if the antibiotics are the cause of coagulopathy or the severity of illness, hepatic or renal function, nutritional status, or oncologic/hematologic diseases; concomitant use of additional coagulopathy pharmacotherapy may influence the coagulation system as well.[41,42]

Antimicrobial drug interactions with warfarin are well known. Most prominent interactions affecting bleeding risk include concomitant use of azole antifungals, even single doses, cephalosporins (second-generation and third-generation), isoniazid, macrolides, metronidazole, rifampin, and sulfonamides. These antimicrobials significantly increase INR by inhibiting warfarin metabolism and warrant close monitoring or empiric decrease in warfarin therapy.[43]

Chemotherapy and Immunosuppressants

Chemotherapy known to cause bone marrow suppression includes methotrexate, 5-fluorouracil, and 6-mercaptopurine. Low platelet counts and low white blood cell counts are of equal concern in chemotherapy patients because decreased platelets may prolong clotting time and decreased white blood cell counts leaves patients at risk for infection. Hematologic effects of methotrexate consist of suppressed hematopoiesis, anemia, pancytopenia, leukopenia, neutropenia, and thrombocytopenia.[44] In addition to myelosuppression, methotrexate may cause acute and chronic hepatotoxicity after prolonged use or a cumulative dose greater than 1.5 g.[45,46] 5-Fluorouracil alters hematologic function via agranulocytosis, anemia, leukopenia, pancytopenia, and thrombocytopenia approximately 9 to 14 days after therapy, with expected recovery by 30 days postdose.[47] 6-Mercaptopurine myelosuppression manifests as anemia, leukopenia, and thrombocytopenia approximately 1 week after therapy in greater than 20% of patients, with the nadir at approximately 14 days post-treatment. Patients with

thiopurine S-methyltransferase deficiency may be at risk of life-threatening myelotoxicity on initiation of 6-mercaptopurine therapy.[48] Additional toxicities seen with 6-mercaptopurine include fatal hepatotoxicity featuring intrahepatic cholestasis and parenchymal cell necrosis. Hepatotoxicity risk is increased with elevated doses greater than 2.5 mg/kg daily; however, hepatic injury may occur with any dose.[47]

Commonly prescribed immunosuppressants (methotrexate, sirolimus, and tacrolimus) are all associated with thrombocytopenia that may lead to prolonged BT. In addition to thrombocytopenia, sirolimus case reports suggested defective fibrin formation and decreased fibrinolysis.[48] Tacrolimus may cause decrease PT and increased INR; however, tacrolimus is more likely to cause renal function abnormalities (acute renal failure and increased serum creatinine) than thrombocytopenia; therefore, caution in CKD patients is warranted.[48]

COAGULATION TESTING

Multiple tests are currently available and in common use. The correlation of these tests to oral hemostasis is still regarded as controversial, but regardless, these tests can help clinicians assess patients' overall status and potential for prolonged bleeding.

Bleeding Time

BT test involves the use of a blood pressure cuff (40 mm Hg) on a selected arm and a standardized incision on the forearm with a scalpel. The incision site is blotted at a specific time schedule and the time the wound takes to stop bleeding is recorded. A normal BT is typically between 3 minutes and 10 minutes and is largely dependent on the method used for BT. This test is referred to as the standard test to determine platelet function. Increased BT can result from abnormal skin and vascular tone; thrombocytopenia; acquired platelet dysfunction, such as aspirin, fibrinolysis, anemia, uremia, liver disease, and von Willebrand factor deficiency; and testing errors.[18] This method is no longer commonly administered due to its invasiveness and lack of reliability.

Prothrombin Time

PT is one of the most commonly used laboratory test used to evaluate patients with hepatic disease. PT measures the extrinsic pathway factors I, II, V, VII, and X by mixing thromboplastin and calcium with citrated plasma. The time it takes to coagulate is then measured with normalized comparisons available (INR). This is a useful test in measuring the level of liver damage and potential for hemostasis. The PT values do not follow a linear relationship to liver function. Studies have shown that 30% to 50% of the liver must be damaged before any appreciable change in PT/INR values.

Platelet Count

The platelet count measures the number of platelets in circulation. Low platelet counts can be due to platelet destruction (alcohol poisoning, liver disease, or sequestration) or decreased production (drugs or leukemia). Normal ranges for platelet counts are 150,000 cells/mm^3 to 450,000 per cells/mm^3. It is generally accepted that platelet counts above 50,000 per cells/mm^3 have a low risk of increased bleeding and, therefore, are a minimal value for elective procedures. Platelet counts between 25,000 per cells/mm^3 and 50,000 per cells/mm^3 have increased risk for postoperative bleeding and elective procedures should be deferred. Only emergent procedures should be performed on patients with platelet counts below 25,000 per cells/mm^3 because they have the potential to be life threatening.[18]

Activated Partial Thromboplastin Time

Activated partial thromboplastin time measures the intrinsic pathway of blood coagulation, including factors II, V, and X. It is particularly useful in evaluating heparin treatment, liver disease, hemophilia, and disseminated intravascular coagulation.[19] In assessing hepatic dysfunction, the PT is more sensitive than the PTT. This is because PT is primarily based on fewer coagulation factors and is particularly dependent on factor VII. Factor VII is of particular relevance because it is the coagulation factor with the shortest half-life and, therefore, the first to become abnormal in hepatic dysfunction.

Thromboelastography

TEG is a viscoelastic hemostatic assay measuring properties of whole blood clot formation under shear stress. TEG displays the interaction of platelets with the coagulation cascade measuring aggregation, clot strength, fibrin cross-linking, and fibrinolysis; however, it does not correlate with standard coagulation assays (PT/INR, aPTT, and anti-Xa).[49] Typically, TEG is indicated in trauma, liver transplantation, cardiac surgery and to guide transfusions. Specific parameters of TEG represent 3 phases of hemostasis: initiation, amplification, and propagation. The initiation phase includes the reaction time (R-value), which correlates to the time to initial fibrin formation. Amplification is represented by kinetics (K), indicating the time taken to achieve clot strength. The angle between the R-value and K (alpha) measures the speed of fibrin cross-linking and clot formation. After formation, the overall stability of the clot is measured by the maximum amplitude (MA) followed by degree of fibrinolysis at 30 minutes (LY30).[49] These TEG values are then used to guide treatment, for example, and increased R-value could indicate use of fresh frozen plasma (FFP) whereas a decreased MA might imply platelets are needed. Patients with acute liver dysfunction and typically cirrhosis maintain normal TEG values. Cirrhotic patients have displayed decreased MA and alpha values, whereas acute liver failure patients may have an increase in MA.[49] End-stage renal disease patients have TEG values suggesting hypercoagulability, as seen with an increase in R-value.[50,51] **Table 2** displays commonly altered TEG values in patients with renal and hepatic dysfunction.

Table 2
Alterations of thromboelastography values in patients with hepatic and renal dysfunction

Impairment	R-value	K	Alpha	MA	LY30
None	5–10 min	1–3 min	53°–72°	50–70 mm	0%–3%
Hepatic[49]					
Acute liver injury/failure	WNL	WNL	↑	↑	WNL
Cirrhosis	WNL	↑	WNL	↓	↑
Renal[50]					
End-stage renal disease	↑	WNL	WNL	WNL	WNL

Abbreviation: WNL, within normal limits.

Data from Stravitz RT. Potential applications of thromboelastography in patients with acute and chronic liver disease. Gastroenterol Hepatol (N Y). 2012;8(8):513–20; and Darlington A, Ferreiro JK, Ueno M, et al. Haemostatic profiles assessed by thromboelastography in patients with end-stage renal disease. Thromb Haemost 2011;106(1):67–74.

IMPLICATIONS FOR ORAL AND MAXILLOFACIAL SURGERY

Patients with systemic diseases pose a risk for increased bleeding as well as hypercoagulation and thrombi formation. A thorough clinical examination with aids from laboratory tests should aid the clinician in determining the coagulation status of a patient. Patients with multiple comorbidities, such as cardiac disease, may be on adjunctive anticoagulants and antiplatelet medications that make the management of these patients more complicated. It has been common practice in the past to alter these anticoagulation and antiplatelet medications by stopping these drugs a set amount of days prior to any elective procedure. There has been no definitive evidence that this practice aids

in improved BT and places patients at increased risk for comorbidities, such as thromboembolism.

Many clinicians choose to bridge patients who are taking anticoagulants in the inpatient setting with heparin or similar medications. This practice also has no sound evidence depicting any benefit but rather the potential for harm. Patients who are bridged from their regular anticoagulant have proved to show an increased risk of major bleeding without any significant reduction in thromboembolism. These practices should be discouraged unless more evidence depicts any advantage in doing thus.

Preoperative assessment and management of hypocoagulable patients are crucial in avoiding increased bleeding events (**Fig. 1**). Most procedures in these patient populations can be

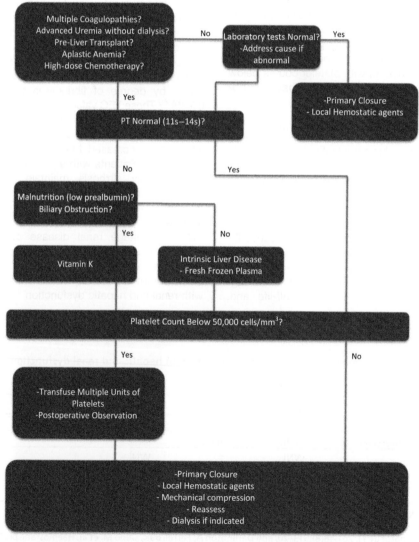

Fig. 1. Preoperative assessment and management of the hypercoagulable patient.

performed safely when properly managed. In cases of a patient with a single coagulopathy, local measures are often sufficient to form hemostasis. These include hemostatic agents, such as oxidized cellulose, tranexamic acid rinses, microfibrillar collogen, astringents, thrombin-soaked gauze, electrocautery, absorbable gelatin sponges, aminocaproic acid, the use of local anesthetics with epinephrine, and primary closure of wounds.

Patients with more advanced single coagulopathies, multiple coagulopathies, platelet counts below 50,000 cells/mm^3, advanced uremia without dialysis, pre–liver transplant status, or aplastic anemia and patients undergoing high-dose chemotherapy (myelosuppressive) are at increased risk for bleeding and require more extensive work-ups for presurgical optimization.

Patients with kidney disease are often optimized for bleeding when their underlying renal disease is properly treated. In management of chronic renal failure, patients are often heparinized for dialysis and therefore are best treated the day after dialysis. It is crucial that these patients are treated in a time appropriate manner because the more time that has passed from patients' last dialysis, the more likely they are to be coagulopathic from their uremia. Baseline laboratory tests are considered beneficial in assessing renal dysfunction status, such as creatinine, GFR, and serum urea nitrogen.

Liver failure patients are often evaluated with a PT test. When evaluating PT results, a small increase in PT time due to liver disease represents a substantial damage to the hepatic system (up to 50%) and does not depict a linear relationship to liver disease.[19] Testing these liver failure patients (complete blood cell count, basic metabolic panel, liver function tests, and PT/INR) preoperatively allows a clinician to determine the underlying cause and potential risk associated with their disease, enabling proper optimization of a patient. Elevated PT times from a hepatic position commonly represents malnutrition, biliary obstruction, or intrinsic liver disease. In cases of malnutrition or biliary obstruction–related coagulopathy, vitamin K should be administered to correct hypoprothrombinemia. The intrinsic liver disease patient often suffers from decreased coagulant production, with increased PT times benefiting from preoperative FFP. For surgical procedures it is common to administer FFP until a goal INR of 2 (INR of 3 for dental extractions[52]) or a PT value that is within 50% of the normal PT is obtained.[53] Platelet counts are also affected in these patients, as discussed previously. When optimizing these patients for surgery, platelet counts should be above 50,000/mL to improve hemostasis in the elective procedure. Patients with platelet counts below 50,000/mL should be given multiple units of platelets, addressing both quantitative and qualitative dysfunction.

After proper assessment and preoperative optimization, attention should be directed at perioperative and postoperative considerations. In hypocoagulable patients, local measures to obtain hemostasis should be performed perioperatively and postoperatively. Postoperative observation is vital in ensuring appropriate hemostasis, including outpatient observation as well as potential hospital admission depending on the severity of the underlying coagulopathy. Medication administration should be carefully considered and dosing may need to be altered, as indicated previously. Medications, such as analgesics and sedatives, have increased duration of action due to the decreased hepatic and renal clearance and should be tailored accordingly.

SUMMARY

Increased BTs and hemostasis is an increasingly complicated and multifactorial process that necessities surgeons who are well informed and up to date on these contributory factors. It is, therefore, prudent that surgeons properly work up patients and obtain all information available prior to any elective procedures. Signs of increased bleeding, such as bruises, family history, systemic diseases, bleeding disorders, surgical history with outcome, and medications, can all alert the surgeon towards potential hemostasis impairment.[19] Consultation with a patient's primary care physician or hematologist is essential, and laboratory testing may be needed for optimal outcomes. With proper work-up and experience, these patients can be cared for effectively and safely.

REFERENCES

1. Violi F, Leo R, Vezza E, et al. Bleeding time in patients with cirrhosis: relation with degree of liver failure and clotting abnormalities. C.A.L.C Group. Coagulation Abnormalities in Cirrhosis Study Group. J Hepatol 1994;20:531–6.
2. Rampino T, Marasà M, Malvezzi PM, et al. Platelet-independent defect in hemostasis associated with sirolimus use. Transplant Proc 2004;36(3):700–2.
3. Peters DH, Fitton A, Plosker GL, et al. Tacrolimus: a review of its pharmacology, and therapeutic potential in hepatic and renal transplantation. Drugs 1993;46:746–94.
4. Tripodi A, Anstee QM, Sogaard KK, et al. Hypercoagulability in cirrhosis: causes and consequences. J Thromb Haemost 2011;9:1713–23.

5. Tripodi A. Hemostasis abnormalities in cirrhosis. Curr Opin Hematol 2015;22:406–12.

6. Lutz J, Menke J, Sollinger D, et al. Haemostasis in chronic kidney disease. Nephrol Dial Transplant 2014;29(1):29–40.

7. Di Minno G, Martinez J, McKean ML, et al. Platelet dysfunction in uremia. Multifaceted defect partially corrected by dialysis. Am J Med 1985;79:552–9.

8. Mezzano D, Tagle R, Panoo O, et al. Hemostatic disorder of uremia: the platelet defect, main determinant of the prolonged bleeding time, is correlated with indices of activation of coagulation and fibrinolysis. Thromb Haemost 1996;76:312–21.

9. Pawlak K, Pawlak D, Mysliwiec M. Oxidative stress effects fibrinolytic system in dialysis uraemic patients. Thromb Res 2006;117:517–22.

10. Pavord S, Myers B. Bleeding and thrombotic complications of kidney disease. Blood Rev 2011;25:271–8.

11. Monreal M, Falga C, Valle R, et al. Venous thromboembolism in patients with renal insufficiency: findings from the RIETE Registry. Am J Med 2006;119:1073–9.

12. Cook DJ, Crowther MA, Meade MO, et al. Prevalence, incidence, and risk factors for venous thromboembolism in medical-surgical intensive care unit patients. J Crit Care 2005;20:309–13.

13. Ocak G, Verduijn M, Vossen CY, et al. Chronic kidney disease stages 1–3 increase the risk of venous thrombosis. J Thromb Haemost 2010;8:2428–35.

14. Shlipak MG, Fried LF, Crump C, et al. Elevations of inflammatory and procoagulant biomarkers in elderly persons with renal insufficiency. Circulation 2003;107:87–92.

15. Pawlak K, Tankiewicz J, Mysliwiec M, et al. Tissue factor/its pathway inhibitor system and kynurenines in chronic kidney disease patients on conservative treatment. Blood Coagul Fibrinolysis 2009;20:590–4.

16. Chu AJ. Tissue factor mediates inflammation. Arch Biochem Biophys 2005;440:123–32.

17. Tomura S, Nakamura Y, Deguchi F, et al. Coagulation and fibrinolysis in patients with chronic renal failure undergoing conservative treatment. Thromb Res 1991;64:81–90.

18. Lockhart PB. Dental management considerations for the patient with acquired coagulopathy. Br Dent J 2003;195:439–45.

19. Dalati MH, Kudsi Z, Koussayer LT, et al. Management of bleeding disorders in the dental practice: managing patients on anticoagulants. Dent Update 2012;39(4):266–70.

20. Hon Y. Dose adjustment in renal and hepatic disease. McGraw Hill Education: Applied Biopharmaceutics & Pharmacokinetics, 7e; 2016.

21. Dabigatran. Lexi-Drugs. [package insert]. Hudson, OH: Lexicomp; Wolters Kluwer Health, Inc. Available at: http://online.lexi.com. Accessed February 18, 2014.

22. Warfarin. Lexi-Drugs. [package insert]. Hudson, OH: Lexicomp; Wolters Kluwer Health, Inc. Available at: http://online.lexi.com. Accessed February 18, 2014.

23. Aspirin. Lexi-Drugs. [package insert]. Hudson, OH: Lexicomp; Wolters Kluwer Health, Inc. Available at: http://online.lexi.com. Accessed February 18, 2014.

24. Rivaroxaban. Lexi-Drugs. [package insert]. Hudson, OH: Lexicomp; Wolters Kluwer Health, Inc. Available at: http://online.lexi.com. Accessed February 18, 2014.

25. Apixiban. Lexi-Drugs. [package insert]. Hudson, OH: Lexicomp; Wolters Kluwer Health, Inc. Available at: http://online.lexi.com. Accessed February 18, 2014.

26. Endoxaban. Lexi-Drugs. [package insert]. Hudson, OH: Lexicomp; Wolters Kluwer Health, Inc. Available at: http://online.lexi.com. Accessed February 18, 2014.

27. Clopidogrel. Lexi-Drugs. [package insert]. Hudson, OH: Lexicomp; Wolters Kluwer Health, Inc. Available at: http://online.lexi.com. Accessed February 18, 2014.

28. Prasugrel. Lexi-Drugs. [package insert]. Hudson, OH: Lexicomp; Wolters Kluwer Health, Inc. Available at: http://online.lexi.com. Accessed February 18, 2014.

29. Ticagrelor. Lexi-Drugs. [package insert]. Hudson, OH: Lexicomp; Wolters Kluwer Health, Inc. Available at: http://online.lexi.com. Accessed February 18, 2014.

30. Armstrong MJ, Gronseth G, Anderson DC, et al. Summary of evidence-based guideline: periprocedural management of antithromboic medications in patients with ischemic cerebrovascular disease: report of the Guideline Development Subcommittee of the American Academy of Neurology. Neurology 2013;80(22):2065–9.

31. Poulsen BK, Grove EL, Husted SE. New oral anticoagulants; a review of the literature with particular emphasis on patients with impaired renal function. Drugs 2012;72(13):1739–53.

32. Kaatz S, Kouides PA, Garcia DA, et al. Guidance on the emergent reversal of oral thrombin and factor Xa inhibitors. Am J Hematol 2012;87(Suppl 1):S141–5.

33. Levi M, Eerenberg E, Kamphuisen PW. Bleeding risk and reversal strategies for old and new anticoagulants and antiplatelet agents. J Thromb Haemost 2011;9(9):1705–12.

34. Siegal DM, Cumutte JT, Connolly SJ, et al. Andexanet alfa for the reversal of factor Xa activity. N Engl J Med 2015;373:2413–24.

35. Pollack CV, Reilly PA, Eikelboom J, et al. Idarucizumab for dabigatran reversal. N Engl J Med 2015;373(6):511–20.

36. Boehringer Ingelheim. Pradaxa® (dabigatran etexilate mesylate) capsules prescribing information. Ridgefield (CT): Boehringer Ingelheim; 2014.

37. You JJ, Singer DE, Howard PA, et al. Antithrombotic therapy in atrial fibrillation. Chest 2012;141(suppl): e531s–75s.

38. Janssen. Xarelto® (rivaroxaban) oral tablets prescribing information. Titusville (NJ): Janssen; 2014.

39. Bristol-Myers Squibb. Eliquis® (apixaban) oral tablets prescribing information. Princeton (NJ): Bristol-Myers Squibb; 2014.

40. Daiichi Sankyo. Inc. Savaysa® (edoxaban) oral tablets prescribing information. Parsippany (NJ): Daiichi Sankyo; 2015.

41. Hirsh J, Fuster V. Guide to anticoagulant therapy. Part 2: oral anticoagulants. American Heart Association. Circulation 1994;89:1469–80.

42. Bandrowsky T, Vorono AA, Borris TJ, et al. Amoxicillin-related postextraction bleeding in an anticoagulated patient with tranexamic acid rinses. Oral Surg Oral Med Oral Pathol Oral Radiol Endod 1996;82:610–2.

43. Holbrook AM, Pereira JA, Labiris R, et al. Systematic overview of warfarin and its drug and food interactions. Arch Intern Med 2005;165:1095–106.

44. Bedford Laboratories. Methotrexate for injection prescribing information. Bedford (OH): Bedford Laboratories; 2012.

45. Gilbert SC, Klintmalm G, Menter A, et al. Methotrexate-induced cirrhosis requiring liver transplantation in three patients with psoriasis: a word of caution in light of the expanding use of this "steroid-sparing" agent. Arch Intern Med 1990;150: 889–91.

46. Kevat S, Ahern M, Hall P. Hepatotoxicity of methotrexate in rheumatic diseases. Med Toxicol Adverse Drug Exp 1988;3:197–208.

47. Teva Parenteral Medicines Inc. Adrucil® (fluorouracil) injection prescribing information. Irvine (CA): Teva Parenteral Medicines Inc; 2007.

48. Teva Pharmaceuticals. Purinethol® (mercaptopurine) tablets prescribing information. Sellersville (PA): Teva Pharmaceuticals; 2011.

49. Stravitz RT. Potential applications of thromboelastography in patients with acute and chronic liver disease. Gastroenterol Hepatol (N Y) 2012;8(8): 513–20.

50. Darlington A, Ferreiro JK, Ueno M, et al. Haemostatic profiles assessed by thromboelastography in patients with end-stage renal disease. Thromb Haemost 2011;106(1):67–74.

51. Holloway DS, Vagher JP, Caprini JA, et al. Thromboelastography of blood from subjects with chronic renal failure. Thromb Res 1987;45(6):817–25.

52. Douglas LR, Douglass JB, Sieck JO, et al. Oral management of the patient with end-stage liver disease and the liver transplant patient. Oral Surg Oral Med Oral Pathol Oral Radiol Endod 1998;86:55–64.

53. Alquahtani SA, Fouad TR, Lee SS. Cirrhotic cardiomyopathy. Semin Liver Dis 2008;28:59–69.

Platelet Abnormalities in the Oral Maxillofacial Surgery Patient

Ehlie K. Bruno, DDS[a], Jeffrey D. Bennett, DMD[b],*

KEYWORDS

- Platelets • Immune-mediated thrombocytopenias • Drug-induced thrombocytopenias
- Congenital thrombocytopenias • Acquired thrombocytopenias • Thrombocytosis

KEY POINTS

- Platelet abnormalities result from a wide range of congenital and acquired conditions, which may be known or unknown to patients presenting for oral maxillofacial surgery.
- It is critical to obtain a thorough history, including discussion of any episodes of bleeding or easy bruising, to potentially discern patients with an underlying platelet disorder.
- If patients indicate a positive history, preoperative laboratory studies are indicated, with potential referral or consultation with a hematologist.
- Appropriate preoperative planning may reduce the risk of bleeding associated with platelet dysfunction, potentially avoiding serious perioperative and postoperative complications.

INTRODUCTION

Platelets have multiple functions involving a complex spectrum of processes from hemostasis to thrombosis. Platelet abnormalities have a multifactorial cause when encountered in patients presenting for oral and maxillofacial surgery in both the inpatient and the outpatient environments. It is essential to have an understanding of the physiologic mechanisms underlying platelet disorders in order to effectively manage patients and reduce potential surgical complications within this heterogeneous population. This article provides an overview of platelet physiology and platelet dysfunction, including thrombocytopenia and thrombocytosis.

PHYSIOLOGY OF NORMAL PLATELETS

Platelets are small, nonnucleated cells derived from precursor proplatelets produced by megakaryocytes found in bone marrow. A normal platelet concentration within the blood is between 150,000 and 450,000 cells per microliter. The typical duration of platelet circulation within the human vascular system is approximately 10 days. Platelets are supported by multiple regulators including nitrogen monoxide and prostacyclin.[1] Healthy endothelium is essential in contributing to this passive state, because it provides a physical barrier between the circulating platelets and extrinsic activators contained within the walls of the vessel. These extrinsic regulators serve to downregulate platelet responsiveness, preventing inappropriate activation in the passive state. After vascular injury occurs, platelets are the primary cellular component involved in the hemostatic response in an effort to reduce hemorrhage.

The hemostatic response is commonly modeled triphasically as platelet initiation, extension, and stabilization. During initiation, circulating platelets adhere to von Willebrand factor at the site of injury, forming a monolayer. This monolayer of platelets is

[a] Indiana University, Indianapolis, IN, USA; [b] Division of Oral and Maxillofacial Surgery, Roudebush VA Medical Center, Indianapolis, IN, USA
* Corresponding author.
E-mail address: jb2omfs@gmail.com

Oral Maxillofacial Surg Clin N Am 28 (2016) 473–480
http://dx.doi.org/10.1016/j.coms.2016.06.001
1042-3699/16/$ – see front matter Published by Elsevier Inc.

subsequently activated by collagen complexes. Additional platelets are recruited and adhere to the monolayer during the extension phase. Throughout this phase, platelet storage granules are released. The granules contain additional von Willebrand factor. G protein–coupled receptors on these recruited platelets are activated by thrombin, thromboxane A2, adenosine diphosphate, and epinephrine. Once activated, a cascade of events occurs, ultimately leading to platelet aggregation via activation of integrin $\alpha_{IIb}\beta_3$. von Willebrand factor, fibrinogen, and fibrin use the integrin $\alpha_{IIb}\beta_3$ found on the surface of platelets to create crosslinking.[1] The final component of the hemostatic response is known as stabilization. Stabilization occurs partially by increasing intracellular platelet signaling, thus preventing preemptive dissolution. These events lead to the creation of a newly formed fibrin crosslinked thrombus at the site of vascular injury. The newly formed thrombus is capable of withstanding the forces generated by arterial blood flow.

PHYSIOLOGIC PATHWAYS OF THROMBOCYTOPENIA

Thrombocytopenia is defined as a decrease in total platelet count of less than 150,000 platelets per microliter of blood. Thrombocytopenia may be further classified as mild (100,000–150,000 platelets per microliter), moderate (50,000–100,000 platelets per microliter), or severe (<50,000 platelets per microliter). Mechanisms underlying thrombocytopenia can be divided into 4 categories. These categories include increased platelet destruction, decreased platelet production, platelet sequestration, and thrombocytopenia secondary to hemodilutional effects.

Platelet destruction may be caused by autoimmune disorders, which lead to an overall decrease in the lifespan of circulating platelets. Autoimmune disorders may simultaneously blunt the regulatory response of bone marrow to increase platelet production in light of increased destruction, resulting in thrombocytopenia. Platelet destruction also occurs when platelets are physically damaged. Platelet destruction occurs primarily by the following 3 methods: the presence of damaged microvasculature with multiple thrombi, inappropriate platelet activation by proinflammatory cytokines and thrombin, or physical contact with artificial surfaces. Patients with thrombotic thrombocytopenic purpura, low-platelet syndrome of pregnancy, and hemolytic uremic syndrome have damage intrinsic to the microvasculature. Patients with disseminated intravascular coagulation, abnormal vascular surfaces secondary to cardiac

valve replacement, aneurysms, and vascular malformations may have a propensity for platelet destruction secondary to inappropriate activation as described above. Artificial surfaces involving cardiopulmonary bypass, intra-aortic balloon pumps, or ventricular assist devices are known to cause structural damage also leading to thrombocytopenia.

As described previously, platelets are produced by megakaryocytes contained within the bone marrow. Pathologic processes affecting the maturation or differentiation of these cells can result in decreased production of platelets, with even greater potentially devastating effects on overall hematopoiesis.

Thrombocytopenia secondary to platelet sequestration also occurs in the clinical setting of hypersplenism. Nearly 30% of platelets are stored in a healthy spleen; however, in cases of splenomegaly, this percentage increases. This splenic-mediated pathologic process ultimately leads to platelet destruction. However, in thrombocytopenia secondary to splenomegaly, the total platelet count typically remains greater than 20,000 platelets per microliter, and significant hemostatic disorders are generally absent.[2]

In addition, thrombocytopenia may be secondary to hemodilutional effects in patients receiving large amounts of fluids without transfusion of platelets. The platelet count can decrease by as much as 50% due to hemodilution when 10 to 12 units of packed red blood cells are rapidly transfused.[2]

Although rare, in consideration of the oral maxillofacial surgeon is the phenomenon of pseudothrombocytopenia, also known as spurious thrombocytopenia. Pseudothrombocytopenia represents an event in which platelet clumping occurs ex vivo, typically in a laboratory setting. It is common practice to add a calcium chelator such as EDTA to a blood sample for anticoagulation effects during laboratory processing. The calcium chelator modifies the response of circulating antiplatelet antibodies targeting platelet surface glycoproteins, resulting in clumping. Automated blood counters fail to recognize these aggregates as platelets, leading to an erroneously low platelet count. Occasionally, the aggregates are further misidentified based on size as neutrophils, resulting in a pseudoleukocytosis. However, this abnormal platelet clumping is recognized in a review of the peripheral blood smear. If clumping is present, a second blood sample may be obtained using alternative anticoagulants such as a citrate or heparin; this usually produces a more accurate platelet count. It is estimated that pseudothrombocytopenia occurs within less than 0.3% of the population without any known pathologic sequelae or clinical significance.[2]

CLINICAL EVALUATION OF PATIENTS WITH THROMBOCYTOPENIA

In patients with known medical comorbidities suggestive of a potential coagulopathy, the presence of a platelet disorder should be investigated before surgical treatment. A complete blood count and evaluation of a peripheral smear should be obtained. However, in patients without known coexisting disease, a detailed family history and personal history may warrant additional workup. All surgical patients should be evaluated for a family history of thrombocytopenia. Previous episodes of bleeding or bruising should be discussed preoperatively; this may indicate a possible congenital or acquired condition. Any previous incidental laboratory findings of thrombocytopenia should also be reviewed. Although patients may present asymptomatically or with mild symptoms before surgery, significant morbidity may result from a procedure if appropriate precautions are not established. Many clinical scenarios may warrant consultation, referral, and/or patient management by a board-certified hematologist.

IMMUNE-MEDIATED THROMBOCYTOPENIAS

Primary immune thrombocytopenia is a heterogeneous group of autoimmune disorders that lead to thrombocytopenia due to decreased platelet production and increased platelet clearance.[3] Primary immune thrombocytopenia, formerly known as idiopathic thrombocytopenia purpura (ITP), comprises approximately 80% of immune-mediated cases overall.[4] Autoantibodies are conventionally considered to be the preeminent process underlying platelet destruction by binding to platelet antigens. Specific targets of the autoantibodies are variable. Some autoantibodies recognize a single glycoprotein, whereas others have the capability of recognizing multiple platelet antigens. However, only approximately 60% of patients with primary immune thrombocytopenia will have detectable autoantibodies.[4] Patients without known autoantibodies may have additional processes of platelet destruction and/or decreased testing sensitivity.

Destructive T-cell activity has also been implicated in primary immune thrombocytopenia. Autoantibodies have been shown to have somatic mutations, which is traditionally indicative of a T-cell–mediated response. Abnormal T-cell activity continues to be researched in effort to have a more comprehensive understanding of the underlying pathophysiology.

Secondary immune thrombocytopenia often arises from persistent infections or other coexisting disease. Because of multiple underlying causes, secondary immune thrombocytopenia has widely variable responses to treatment. In most cases involving acute immune thrombocytopenia of childhood, most children have a known preceding febrile illness. As platelets begin to express viral antigens, antiviral antibodies cross-react and generate autoantibodies against the platelets. Platelets are then destroyed at an increased rate with resultant thrombocytopenia. This clinical condition is typically self-limiting, with most children experiencing resolution in 1 year.

Acute secondary immune thrombocytopenia may also develop after vaccinations against a host of infectious agents, including pneumococcus, *Haemophilus influenzae B*, hepatitis B, varicella-zoster, and measles/mumps/rubella (MMR).[4,5] ITP-MMR develops within 42 days of vaccination, and it is estimated to occur 1 in every 40,000 doses.[3] Although the resultant thrombocytopenia is typically severe, 80% of patients are responsive to treatment within 2 months.[4] After vaccination-induced thrombocytopenia, patients may continue to receive all recommended vaccinations when the ITP stabilizes or is in remission.

A growing body of evidence indicates specific infectious agents are associated with developing secondary immune thrombocytopenia. *Helicobacter pylori* infections have been implicated in secondary immune thrombocytopenia, as platelet counts have improved after infection resolution in certain geographic areas. It is unclear whether resolution of an *H pylori* infection has a substantial impact within the United States and European countries. However, in Japan, treatment of *H pylori* appears to have significant clinical benefit.[3] Cytomegalovirus, varicella-zoster, hepatitis C, and HIV have also led to the development of secondary immune thrombocytopenia.[5]

Several neoplastic processes have been linked to secondary immune thrombocytopenia. Chronic lymphocytic leukemia is the most predominant. Approximately 1% to 5% of patients diagnosed with chronic lymphocytic leukemia develop secondary immune thrombocytopenia.[6] A small prevalence of patients with Hodgkin diseases and large granular T-lymphocyte leukemia may also be at risk for developing secondary immune thrombocytopenia.

Secondary immune thrombocytopenia can develop approximately 7 to 10 days after platelet transfusion. The alloantibodies target transfused platelet antigens, resulting in a severe and potentially fatal clinical condition known as posttransfusion purpura (PTP). PTP is an exceedingly rare transfusion complication with an estimated incidence of 1 in 50,000 to 100,000 transfusions.[7] When more common causes of immune thrombocytopenia have been ruled out in critically ill patients, it is essential to maintain a high level of suspicion of PTP. PTP is a self-limiting condition responsive to treatment if delivered within an appropriate period of time.

TREATMENT MODALITIES FOR IMMUNE THROMBOCYTOPENIA

Patients with immune thrombocytopenia that have a platelet count greater than 30,000 per microliter without severe bleeding rarely require any acute intervention. It is recommended that patients with slightly lower platelet counts ranging from 20,000 to 30,000 per microliter remain under careful observation. Emergent management of patients with platelet counts less than 20,000 per microliter or presenting with significant bleeding may necessitate platelet transfusion. Transfusions are discussed in greater detail in subsequent articles of this publication.

Treatment of immune thrombocytopenia is divided into first-line and second-line therapies involving both medical and surgical management. First-line medical management is based on pharmacotherapy. Corticosteroids are recommended as first-line therapy in an effort to reduce circulating autoantibody levels. Treatment is typically initiated with prednisolone at 4 mg/kg for the shortest amount of time possible up to 4 days.[8] Alternatively, intravenous immunoglobulin G (IgG) as a single dose of 0.8 g/kg clears opsonized platelets and induces a faster response than corticosteroids.[9] However, one must consider the rare but potentially devastating side effects of intravenous IgG. These effects include renal failure, acute hemolysis, and thromboembolic events.[10] An additional first-line therapy also includes intravenous anti-D, which comprises antibodies to the RH factor present on red blood cells. Anti-D IGIV targets red blood cells reactive to the D antigen, which then competes with platelets for sequestration in the spleen. Anti-D IGIV may be administered at 75 μg/kg over 3 to 5 minutes.[8] Successful remission of immune thrombocytopenia occurs when patients can maintain a platelet count of 100,000 per microliter or more without pharmacologic management. Unfortunately, this is only achieved in approximately 20% of patients with this clinical condition.[3]

Patients who fail first-line medical management may pose a significant challenge. More than 10 second-line therapies exist, with no comparative trials of these various treatments.[11] For decades, the standard approach to second-line treatment in patients with immune thrombocytopenia has been surgical management. Splenectomies have provided the highest cure rate, with 60% to 70% in remission after 5 years.[11] Utilization of the laparoscopic approach and perioperative thromboprophylaxis has resulted in reduced morbidity and potentially decreased mortality. However, despite the sustainable remission rate, surgical options are invasive, and postoperative complications, including sepsis, have occurred. With promising responses to second-line pharmacotherapy involving Rituximab, physicians may elect for alternative approaches.

Rituxamab is a monoclonal antibody that targets the CD20 antigen on B lymphocytes. This drug reduces circulating autoantibodies by producing a quantitative reduction of B cells. The standard treatment regimen of low-dose Rituxamab consists of 375 mg/m^2 every 7 days for 4 weeks.[12] Complete response with Rituxamab has been demonstrated in 40% of patients after 12 months, with 20% persistently responding at 3 to 5 years.[11] Additional options for second-line pharmacotherapy include immunosuppressive therapy and Dapsone. These therapies are widely used in several countries outside of the United States. Immunosuppressive therapy targeting T-cell function can be initiated with azathioprine, cyclophosphamide, and cyclosporine.[9] Dapsone is a sulfonamide-containing antibiotic that has demonstrated a reversal of thrombocytopenia in approximately 50% of patients.[13] Treatment regimens may vary slightly, although therapy is typically initiated with 100 mg/d for 30 days and subsequently tapered.[13]

DRUG-INDUCED ANTIPLATELET ACTIVITY AND THROMBOCYTOPENIAS

Salicylate is one the most widely used nonsteroidal anti-inflammatory drugs due to a variety of pharmacologic effects, including anti-inflammatory, antineoplastic, antiatherosclerotic, and immunosuppressive functions.[14] Salicylate itself does not display any inhibitory properties of cyclo-oxygenase-1 (COX-1)-dependent platelet activity.[15] In vivo, aspirin is rapidly deacylated and converted back to salicylate in the circulation. This property is attributable to the short half-life of approximately 20 minutes.[15] Despite the short half-life, the acetylated version of salicylate, aspirin, does exert additional cardioprotective effects. Aspirin prevents myocardial infarction and ischemic stroke by irreversibly inhibiting COX-1. Inhibition of COX-1 subsequently prevents the formation of thromboxane A2, adversely affecting platelet aggregation. Many oral maxillofacial surgery patients on chronic aspirin therapy will display the effects of dysfunctional platelet aggregation. It is prudent to consider this increased risk of postoperative bleeding when evaluating patients. Multiple other pharmacologic agents exerting antiplatelet activity are discussed in other articles within this volume.

Drug-induced thrombocytopenia may be caused by non-immune-mediated processes leading to myelosuppression, as in the case of chemotherapeutic drugs. More commonly, however, prescription medications, over-the-counter supplements, or food items trigger immune-mediated pathways. Sudden, severe thrombocytopenia may occur, often with platelet counts of less than 20,000 per microliter.[16] If a thorough history is not obtained from the patient, a true case of drug-induced thrombocytopenia may easily be misdiagnosed as immune thrombocytopenia or undetermined. Antiplatelet antibodies from the offending agent typically develop within 1 to 2 weeks of drug administration. However, the potential to develop drug-induced thrombocytopenia exists after intermittent, long-term exposure.[16] Significant morbidity and potential mortality secondary to coagulopathy may result if the underlying etiologic agent is not promptly identified and removed. Quinine, a basic amine found in tonic water, and quinidine are among the highest reported causative agents. Several other offending agents include trimethoprim/sulfamethoxazole (Bactrim, Septra), vancomycin, carbamazepine (Tegretol), acetaminophen, hydrochlorothiazide, and heparin.[16] Because drug-induced thrombocytopenia only occurs in the presence of the agent and persists only with continual administration, prompt resolution occurs after removal of the drug. Patients display improvement generally within 48 hours, and platelet counts normalize within 7 to 14 days.[2]

In the unique case of heparin-induced thrombocytopenia, antiplatelet antibodies lead to aberrantly increased platelet activation. Subsequent thrombosis occurs within 5 to 14 days of heparin administration.[17] With multiple thrombi circulating in the vasculature, the total platelet count decreases, thus causing thrombocytopenia. Although heparin-induced thrombocytopenia rarely results in significant bleeding, the presence of multiple thrombi can have potentially devastating effects.

CONGENITAL THROMBOCYTOPENIAS

Patients presenting with a history of bruising or significant bleeding, a family history significant for thrombocytopenia, or an incidental laboratory finding of thrombocytopenia may warrant workup for congenital thrombocytopenia. Congenital thrombocytopenias encompass numerous syndromes, typically presenting with an early onset. Because of the heterogeneous nature of these disorders, there is significant variation in bleeding tendencies ranging from extremely mild to potentially fatal bleeding episodes. These conditions as a whole are rare and may be genetically transmitted as autosomal-dominant, autosomal-recessive, or X-linked disorders.

Several more commonly known autosomal-dominant thrombocytopenias include MYH9-related diseases, platelet-type von Willebrand disease, and Paris-Trousseau syndrome.

MYH9-related diseases occur secondary to more than 40 identified mutations in the MYH9 gene. MYH9 codes for the nonmuscle myosin heavy chain IIA, located on chromosome 22q12-13.[18] These diseases encompass multiple disorders, including Epstein syndrome, Sebastian syndrome, and Fechtner syndrome. The May-Hegglin anomaly is also related, presenting with leukocyte inclusion bodies (Döhle bodies) and macrothrombocytopenia. With the May-Hegglin anomaly, mean platelet counts range from 20,000 to 130,000 per microliter. MYH9-related diseases present with variable nephropathy, cataracts, and sensorineural hearing loss.[7,19] Some patients remain asymptomatic, although bleeding tendencies are generally mild to moderate. In rare cases, severe bleeding episodes, including intracranial hemorrhage, have been reported.

Platelet-type von Willebrand disease was identified in 1982. This condition results from mutations in the GP1BA gene, which causes defects in platelet surface glycoprotein Ib.[18] Thrombocytopenia occurs after the surface glycoprotein pathologically binds to plasma von Willebrand factor, reducing the quantities of circulating platelets. The clinical manifestations are similar to type 2B von Willebrand disease, which occurs secondary to a mutation within the von Willebrand protein. However, it is essential to differentiate between these disorders due to divergent therapeutic protocols. Treatment of platelet-type von Willebrand disease primarily consists of platelet transfusion, whereas factor VIII infusion is indicated for type 2B von Willebrand disease.

In 1993, an additional form of macrothrombocytopenia known as Paris-Trousseau syndrome was identified. This disorder presents as a mild-to-moderate thrombocytopenia secondary to a subpopulation of platelets, known as Paris-Trousseau platelets. These dysfunctional platelets contain giant α granules. When Paris-Trousseau platelets are stimulated by thrombin after vascular insult, the contents of the α granules are erroneously retained within the platelet, preventing formation of a normal thrombus. In this disorder, the bone marrow also demonstrates an increase in immature megakaryocytes, indicating significant dysmegakaryopoiesis. Paris-Trousseau syndrome may be an isolated clinical condition or present concurrently with Jacobsen syndrome, both of which are associated with a chromosomal deletion at the distal portion of 11q23.[19] Patients with Jacobsen syndrome have macrothrombocytopenia along with facial dysmorphism, mental retardation, syndactyly, trigonocephaly, cardiac defects, and gastrointestinal and renal abnormalities.

Autosomal-recessive thrombocytopenias of note include Bernard-Soulier syndrome (BSS), chromosome 22q11.2 deletion syndrome, Glanzmann thrombasthenia, gray platelet syndrome, and thrombocytopenia with absent radius syndrome (TARS).

First described in 1948, BSS is an exceedingly rare disorder, with an estimated prevalence of less than one per million.[20] BSS is characterized by macrothrombocytopenia and prolonged bleeding time. Bleeding time is increased secondary to defects in the platelet surface receptor for von Willebrand factor.[21] In BSS, platelets are unable to adhere to blood vessels after vascular insult; this produces the common clinical manifestations, including gingival bleeding, epistaxis, menorrhagia, and mucocutaneous purpura.[21]

Chromosome 22q11.2 deletion syndrome, also known as DiGeorge syndrome or velocardiofacial syndrome, has an extensive variety of phenotypic features. Cardiac abnormalities, velopharyngeal insufficiency, delayed speech, and immunodeficiency are among the more prevalent findings.[22] In more than 90% of cases, the deleted portion of chromosome 22q11.2 contains the GP1BB gene, which encodes for a platelet surface receptor subunit.[18] However, a portion of the other chromosome remains intact and thus unaffected. Patients are essentially heterozygous carriers, typically manifesting with a more mild presentation of thrombocytopenia.

Glanzmann thrombasthenia occurs secondary to defects in integrin $\alpha_{IIb}\beta_3$. With dysfunctional integrin, platelet adhesion to proteins including fibrinogen during clot formation is inhibited.[23] Platelet spreading via collagen interaction is also impaired. Glanzmann thrombasthenia produces variable but potentially significant bleeding.[23]

Gray platelet syndrome is characterized by large, grayish-colored platelets without α granules. Gray platelet syndrome is primarily an autosomal-recessive disorder, although autosomal-dominant and X-linked inheritance has been reported.[24] This qualitative, agranular defect leads to moderate thrombocytopenia with typically mild-to-moderate bleeding potential.

TARS is a unique autosomal-recessive disorder with unclear genetic underpinnings. Severe thrombocytopenia is present at birth and demonstrates spontaneous improvement after the first 12 months of life. Additional clinical features of TARS include absence of radii while retaining normal thumbs, along with potential facial deformities, cardiac defects, and renal abnormalities.

Congenital thrombocytopenias with X-linked inheritance include Wiskott-Aldrich syndrome (WAS) and X-linked thrombocytopenia. WAS represents a severe immune dysregulation. Mutation of the WAS gene on chromosome Xp11.22-p11.23 causes resultant macrothrombocytopenia.[18] Additional clinical manifestations include recurrent infections, T-cell deficiency, lymphoproliferative disease, and eczema. A milder condition known as X-linked thrombocytopenia is an allelic variant of WAS, presenting with eczema and a decreased platelet count without any additional immunodeficiency.

ACQUIRED THROMBOCYTOPENIAS

Although a significant amount of cases of thrombocytopenia occur in the context of autoimmune, pharmacologic, and congenitally mediated causes, significantly low platelet counts may be acquired secondary to liver dysfunction, nutritional deficiencies, and renal dysfunction. In alcoholic cirrhosis of the liver, chronic thrombocytopenia is typically a result of portal hypertension and splenomegaly, which in turn causes splenic sequestration. The resultant thrombocytopenia may appear isolated or as a component of pancytopenia. Alcoholism also directly causes bone marrow suppression, which may decrease platelet production. Although there are multiple causes of thrombocytopenia in patients with chronic liver disease, resultant coagulopathies are generally severe.

Although folate deficiency is a common comorbidity of alcoholism, folate and vitamin B12 deficiencies independently inhibit purine synthesis. Inhibition may cause severe thrombocytopenia in the context of pancytopenia and megaloblastosis. In the case of an isolated nutritional deficiency, appropriate repletion of folate and vitamin B12 will rapidly restore platelet counts.

Patients with chronic renal failure may demonstrate hematologic sequelae, including anemia and thrombocytopenia. Decreased platelet counts are frequently encountered, although the exact mechanism remains controversial.[25] When treating patients with known or suspected hepatic, nutritional, or renal deficiencies, one must consider the potential for a secondary coagulopathy.

THROMBOCYTOSIS

Thrombocytosis is a relatively common laboratory finding that may warrant referral for additional investigation. Thrombocytosis occurs when there is an overproduction of platelets increasing the total platelet count to greater than 450,000 platelets per microliter. Although a typical adult platelet count is less, approximately 2.5% of the population will naturally have a platelet count greater than 450,000 per microliter without any associated abnormality.[26]

Hereditary thrombocythemia, also known as familial thrombocytosis, is a rare autosomal-dominant disorder involving megakaryocyte proliferation. It is caused by several identified genetic mutations, including gain-of-function mutations in thrombopoietin. The MPL gene encoding for the thrombopoietin receptor has also been implicated in the pathogenesis, leading to coagulopathy.[27]

Most elevated platelet counts are a result of acquired conditions, including multiple myeloproliferative disorders rather than congenital causes. Although discussion of myeloproliferative disorders is beyond the scope of discussion, it is imperative to consider platelet abnormalities in patients with neoplastic diseases involving bone marrow.

SUMMARY

Platelet abnormalities result from a wide range of congenital and acquired conditions, which may be known or unknown to patients presenting for oral maxillofacial surgery. It is critical to obtain a thorough history, including discussion of any episodes of bleeding or easy bruising to potentially discern patients with an underlying platelet disorder. If patients indicate a positive history, preoperative laboratory studies are indicated, with potential referral or consultation with a hematologist. Appropriate preoperative planning may reduce the risk of bleeding associated with platelet dysfunction, potentially avoiding serious perioperative and postoperative complications.

REFERENCES

1. Brass LF, Tomaiuolo M, Stalker TJ. Harnessing the platelet signaling network to produce an optimal hemostatic response. Hematol Oncol Clin North Am 2013;27(3):381–409.
2. Wong EY, Rose MG. Why does my patient have thrombocytopenia? Hematol Oncol Clin North Am 2012;26(2):231–52.
3. Kashiwagi H, Tomiyama Y. Pathophysiology and management of primary immune thrombocytopenia. Int J Hematol 2013;98(1):24–33.
4. Cines DB, Bussel JB, Liebman HA, et al. The ITP syndrome: pathogenic and clinical diversity. Blood 2009;113(26):6511–21.
5. Kistangari G, McCrae KR. Immune thrombocytopenia. Hematol Oncol Clin North Am 2013;27(3):495–520.
6. Zent CS, Kay NE. Autoimmune complications in chronic lymphocytic leukemia (CLL). Best Pract Res Clin Haematol 2010;23(1):47–59.
7. Padhi P, Parihar GS, Stepp J, et al. Post-transfusion purpura: a rare and life-threatening aetiology of thrombocytopenia. BMJ Case Rep 2013;2013:1–3.
8. Krishnegowda M, Rajashekaraiah V. Platelet disorders: an overview. Blood Coagul Fibrinolysis 2015;26(5):479–91.
9. Warrier R, Chauhan A. Management of immune thrombocytopenic purpura: an update. Ochsner J 2012;12(3):221–7.
10. Berger M. Adverse effects of IgG therapy. J Allergy Clin Immunol Pract 2013;1(6):558–66.
11. Ghanima W, Godeau B, Cines DB, et al. How I treat immune thrombocytopenia: the choice between splenectomy or a medical therapy as a second-line treatment. Blood 2012;120(5):960–9.
12. Zaja F, Battista ML, Pirrotta MT, et al. Lower dose rituximab is active in adults patients with idiopathic thrombocytopenic purpura. Haematologica 2008;93(6):930–3.
13. Vancine-Califani SM, De Paula EV, Ozelo MC, et al. Efficacy and safety of dapsone as a second-line treatment in non-splenectomized adults with immune thrombocytopenic purpura. Platelets 2008;19(7):489–95.
14. Kazama I, Baba A, Endo Y, et al. Salicylate inhibits thrombopoiesis in rat megakaryocytes by changing the membrane micro-architecture. Cell Physiol Biochem 2015;35(6):2371–82.
15. Wu KK. Aspirin and salicylate: an old remedy with a new twist. Circulation 2000;102(17):2022–3.
16. Chong BH, Choi PY, Khachigian L, et al. Drug-induced immune thrombocytopenia. Hematol Oncol Clin North Am 2013;27(3):521–40.
17. Lee GM, Arepally GM. Heparin-induced thrombocytopenia. Hematology Am Soc Hematol Educ Program 2013;2013:668–74.

18. Kumar R, Kahr WHA. Congenital thrombocytopenia: clinical manifestations, laboratory abnormalities, and molecular defects of a heterogeneous group of conditions. Hematol Oncol Clin North Am 2013; 27(3):465–94.

19. Geddis AE, Kaushansky K. Inherited thrombocytopenias: toward a molecular understanding of disorders of platelet production. Curr Opin Pediatr 2004;16(1):15–22.

20. Diz-Kücükkaya R, López JA. Inherited disorders of platelets: membrane glycoprotein disorders. Hematol Oncol Clin North Am 2013;27(3):613–27.

21. Kunishima S, Kamiya T, Saito H, et al. Genetic abnormalities of Bernard-Soulier syndrome. Int J Hematol 2002;76(4):319–27.

22. Lawrence S, McDonald-McGinn DM, Zackai E, et al. Thrombocytopenia in patients with chromosome 22q11.2 deletion syndrome. J Pediatr 2003;143(2): 277–8.

23. Nurden AT, Nurden P. Congenital platelet disorders and understanding of platelet function. Br J Haematol 2014;165(2):165–78.

24. Nurden AT, Nurden P. Inherited disorders of platelet function: selected updates. J Thromb Haemost 2015;13(Suppl 1):S2–9.

25. Dorgalaleh A, Mahmudi M, Tabibian S, et al. Anemia and thrombocytopenia in acute and chronic renal failure. Int J Hematol Oncol Stem Cell Res 2013; 7(4):34–9.

26. Sulai NH, Tefferi A. Why does my patient have thrombocytosis? Hematol Oncol Clin North Am 2012; 26(2):285–301.

27. Wiestner A, Padosch SA, Ghilardi N, et al. Hereditary thrombocythaemia is a genetically heterogeneous disorder: exclusion of TPO and MPL in two families with hereditary thrombocythaemia. Br J Haematol 2000;110(1): 104–9.

Hemophilia
What the Oral and Maxillofacial Surgeon Needs to Know

Julie Ann Smith, DDS, MD, MCR

KEYWORDS

- Hemophilia • Hemophilia inhibitors • Factor VIII deficiency • Factor IX deficiency
- Bleeding disorders • Factor VIII bypass agents

KEY POINTS

- The most significant complication of hemophilia management is the development of inhibitors, which may impact surgical care.
- Acquired hemophilia A is a rare, potential cause of unexpected bleeding, and should be considered whenever a patient presents with unexpected postoperative bleeding.
- Replacement factor administered preoperatively in severe hemophiliacs should be administered within 20 minutes of the start of the procedure owing to the short half-lives of factor replacement.
- From a surgical perspective, hemophiliacs should be managed differently from the typical nonhemophiliac patient with alteration in local anesthetic technique, use of antifibrinolytic therapy, and more intensive follow-up.

INTRODUCTION

Of congenital coagulation factor deficiencies, hemophilia A and hemophilia B are among the most common, and will be encountered in the oral and maxillofacial surgery office. Both are X-linked disorders resulting in a deficiency of either factor VIII (hemophilia A) or factor IX (hemophilia B). Hemophilia A occurs in approximately 1:5000 male births and hemophilia B occurs in approximately 1:30,000 male births. There is no specific geographic or racial predilection. Classic symptoms include soft tissue bleeding and hemarthroses, which can result in debilitating arthropathy. Clinically, hemophilia A and B are indistinguishable. Certainly, any type of bleeding is possible, but 3 key areas where bleeding may be fatal are of particular concern in the hemophiliac: intracranial (leading cause of death in these patients), into the iliopsoas muscle, and in the neck and retropharyngeal space, which may impact the airway.[1] In general, the severity of clinical expression is related to level of factor activity in the plasma and is classified as mild (factor activity 5–40%), moderate (factor activity 1–5%), or severe (factor activity <1%). Normal factor level ranges from 50% to 100%.[2] Patients with mild hemophilia typically will not have spontaneous bleeding, and will only have bleeding in response to trauma, surgical procedures, or dental extractions. Those with moderate hemophilia may experience excess bleeding after trauma, surgery, or dental extractions and may also sustain joint or muscle bleeding after minor injury. Patients with severe hemophilia may experience spontaneous bleeding into joints and muscles and severe bleeding after injuries or surgery. Within the levels of severity, however, there is variable phenotypic expression. Approximately 10% to 15% of patients with hemophilia A exhibit a less severe phenotype and experience less spontaneous bleeding and consume less factor

Oral and Maxillofacial Surgery, Willamette Dental Group, 405 SE 133rd Avenue, Portland, OR 97233, USA
E-mail address: surgeonchick@hotmail.com

Oral Maxillofacial Surg Clin N Am 28 (2016) 481–489
http://dx.doi.org/10.1016/j.coms.2016.06.006
1042-3699/16/$ – see front matter © 2016 Elsevier Inc. All rights reserved.

concentrates. This heterogeneity is the result of genetics as well as environment, and may also be related to laboratory diagnostic factors.[3]

HISTORICAL PERSPECTIVE

Historical references to hemophilia date back to the second century CE, as evidenced in the Babylonian Talmud, which indicates that if a woman has had her first 2 sons die after circumcision, she is exempt from having the third son circumcised.[4] Modern reports of an inherited bleeding disorder that was passed on from females, but only affected males, were documented in the late 1700s and early 1800s. The term *haemophilia* (literally, "affinity to blood") was first used to describe this disorder in 1828 by German physician Johann Lukas Schonlein and his student, Friedrich Hopff. Haemophilia was known as "the royal disease" because it affected various royal families in England, Germany, Spain, and Russia. The royal disease is believed to have been hemophilia B. Early treatments of hemophilia (in the 1800s) involved blood transfusions, which were often fatal, until the concept of cross-matching was introduced. In 1964, the discovery that cryoprecipitate from thawed frozen plasma contained large concentrations of factor VIII, revolutionized hemophilia management. Sadly, the 1980s brought an era during which thousands of hemophiliacs lost their lives to AIDS as plasma derived clotting factor was contaminated with human immunodeficiency virus. Pasteurization of factor concentrate was introduced in 1981 and, ultimately, all plasma-derived products were manufactured virus free by the end of the 1980s, free from human immunodeficiency virus and hepatitis B and C. Recombinant factors became available in 1992, allowing for mass production of clotting factors. Recent progress has led to the development of bypassing agents used in the management of hemophiliacs with inhibitors as well as the development of immune tolerance therapy to reduce or eliminate inhibitors (more on inhibitors elsewhere in this article).[4,5]

OVERVIEW OF COAGULATION

Upon blood vessel injury, hemostasis occurs via primary and secondary mechanisms. Primary hemostasis involves vascular contraction, platelet adhesion, and the formation of a soft platelet plug. Secondary hemostasis is initiated by the release of tissue factor (TF) and involves a complex coagulation cascade. The goal of secondary hemostasis is to stabilize the platelet plug. The traditional model of the coagulation cascade, divided into intrinsic and extrinsic pathways, is no longer considered absolute and a more cell based model has taken its place.[1,6] The initiating event is the release from injured endothelium of TF. TF combines with factor VII to form TF-factor VIIa, which activates factor X and factor IX to factor Xa and factor IXa. factor Xa combines with factor Va to form prothrombinase, and factor IXa combines with factor VIIIa to form tenase Both prothrombinase and tenase convert factor II (prothrombin) into factor IIa (thrombin), which ultimately converts fibrinogen into fibrin. The initial amount of thrombin formed by this process is actually insufficient, so thrombin begins a feedback process, which activates previous components of the coagulation cascade, including factor V and factor VIII, ultimately propagating the coagulation cascade. Several inhibitors along the way regulate this process, including antithrombin, protein C, protein S, and TF pathway inhibitor (**Fig. 1**).[6]

CONGENITAL HEMOPHILIA

Factor VIII is made in the liver and endothelial cells and functions as a cofactor of factor IXa in the tensae complex (factor IXa–factor VIIIa), which activates factor X to factor Xa. Factor IX is made in the liver and the activated form combines with factor VIIIa forming the tensae complex (activating factor X). Lack of either factor VIII or factor IX leads to decreased thrombin formation, and an inability to form a clot. Both hemophilia A and B are X-linked recessive disorders, making hemophilia much more common in males than females. In hemophilia A, approximately 30% of mutations are de novo, and in hemophilia B, more than 33% of mutations are de novo.[6] Of the inherited clotting disorders, hemophilia A and B are the only ones that are inherited in a sex-linked recessive manner. A father with hemophilia will produce female offspring who are carriers, but no male offspring will be affected. A female carrier has a 50% chance of having a son with hemophilia and a 50% chance of having a daughter who is a carrier. It is important to recognize that up to one-third of hemophilia carriers may have reduced levels of factor VIII or factor IX and may have bleeding issues similar to that seen in mild hemophiliacs.[2,6] For this reason, it is recommended that carriers also undergo measurement of factor activity, especially before becoming a surgical patient, because they may require the same management as a mild hemophiliac.[2]

Most severe hemophiliacs will present with excessive bleeding during the first year of life.

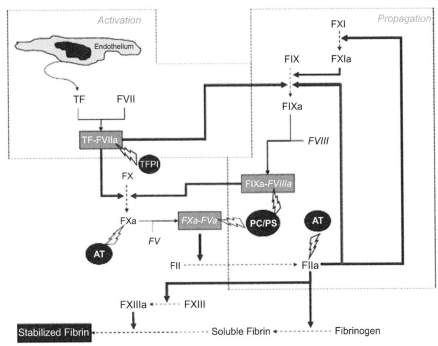

Fig. 1. Overview of the in vivo blood coagulation cascade. AT, antithrombin; F, factor; PC/PS, protein C/protein S; TF, tissue factor. (*From* Lippi G, Franchini M, Montagnana M, et al. Inherited disorders of blood coagulation. Ann Med 2012;44:405–18; with permission.)

Easy bruising and intramuscular hematomas are commonly seen; however, the hallmark of hemophilia is the development of hemarthroses. The joints that are involved in decreasing frequency include the knees, elbows, ankles, shoulders, wrists, and hips.[1] These hemarthroses can predispose the patient to very painful arthropathies and debilitating joint dysfunction, the prevention of which is the basis for prophylactic management of hemophilia. Laboratory findings in hemophilia A and B include a normal prothrombin time, thrombin time, and bleeding time, with an increased prothrombin time (PTT). In a patient with severe hemophilia, the PTT will be 2 to 3 times higher than normal. Further testing is completed to determine the level of factor activity and help categorize the level of disease severity as mild, moderate, or severe (as described in the introduction). A mixing study may be performed in which the hemophiliac's plasma is mixed with a nonhemophiliac's plasma. In a mixing study, the PTT should normalize. If it does not, however, this suggests the presence of an inhibitor (see next section). A Bethesda assay will be performed to further quantify the inhibitor. Other factor deficiencies in addition to factors VIII and IX, which result in an isolated elevation of PTT, include deficiency of factors XI and XII (**Fig. 2**).[6]

INHIBITORS

The most significant complication of modern hemophilia management is the development of inhibitors. Inhibitors are immunoglobulins (IgG), which develop against factor VIII or factor IX and prevent effectiveness of infused factor. Inhibitors are IgG mediated and occur more commonly in severe hemophilia A (≤30% of patients, and 52% by some reports) than in severe hemophilia B (~5% of patients).[7] Although inhibitors are less common in hemophilia B, they put the patient at high risk of severe anaphylaxis and nephrotic syndrome upon administration of factor IX concentrate. Inhibitors are very rare in mild hemophilia, but if they do occur in mild hemophilia, the presence of the inhibitor changes the category of disease to severe.[8] Prophylaxis is believed to reduce the risk of inhibitor development.[7,9] Inhibitors most commonly develop during the first 50 exposures to factor, with a mean age of onset of 1 to 2 years.[1] Some reports indicate that the greatest risk of inhibitor development occurs within the first 20 exposure days.[7] The greatest risk of inhibitor development is associated with severe disease, large gene deletions that result in complete lack of endogenous factor, early age (before 6 months) of factor exposure, and family history of

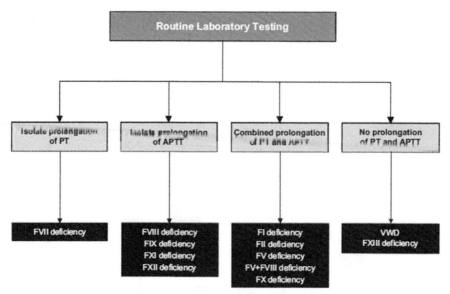

Fig. 2. Abnormalities of routine coagulations tests in patients with inherited coagulation factor (F) disorders. Some cases of von Willebrand disease (VWD) may also present with isolated prolongation of activated partial thromboplastin time (APTT; when low factor VIII levels are also evident). Owren-based prothrombin time (PT) results may be normal in FV deficiency. Primary hemostasis defects such as thrombocytopenias and platelet function disorders should yield normal PT and APTT values. (*From* Lippi G, Franchini M, Montagnana M, et al. Inherited disorders of blood coagulation. Ann Med 2012;44:405–18; with permission.)

inhibitors.[7,9] Ethnicity is also felt to play a role, with increased risk noted in Afro-Caribbeans.[9] Multiple studies on risk factors for inhibitor development have shown conflicting results. Until recently, the studies that examined the question of whether inhibitor development is more likely with exposure to plasma-derived factor VIII or with recombinant factor VIII were not randomized clinical trials.[5] Most nonrandomized studies have suggested that recombinant factor VIII use is more likely to be associated with the development of inhibitors. Recently, an abstract of the only randomized clinical trial (open label) to examine this question (Survey of Inhibitors in Plasma-Product Exposed Toddlers [SIPPET]), was presented.[10] This study has demonstrated a 1.87 higher incidence of inhibitor development after exposure to recombinant factor VIII.

Inhibitors are classified according to inhibitor titer expressed in Bethesda units per milliliter. Patients who have inhibitor titers less than 5 BU/mL have a "low titer" and those with inhibitor titers equal to or greater than 5 BU/mL have a "high titer." Once an inhibitor is present, the response to further factor administration can further stratify the inhibitor severity. If a patient with inhibitors is administrated factor and the titer of the inhibitor does not increase, the patient is said to be a "low responder." If a patient with inhibitors is administered factor and their inhibitor titer quickly increases even higher, they are considered to be a "high responder." The inhibitor titer and level of response to factor are influential in the management of these patients.

Management of inhibitors focuses on treatment of acute bleeds and ultimately, eradication of the inhibitor via immune tolerance induction (ITI). Patients who have low inhibitor titer (<5 BU/mL) who are low responders and who have an acute bleed or need for a surgical procedure are managed with the administration of high doses of either factor VIII (for hemophilia A) or factor IX (for hemophilia B). The use of high doses of factor in these patients should overcome the inhibitor. Patients who have a high titer of inhibitor (≥5 BU/mL) who are high responders require administration of bypassing agents, because even high doses of factor are not sufficient to overcome the inhibitor in these patients. The 2 commercially available bypassing agents are activated prothrombin complex concentrate factor VIII inhibitor bypass agent (APCC FEIBA; usually abbreviated FEIBA) and recombinant activated factor VII (rFVIIa). The management of hemophilia B patients with inhibitors is complicated by the fact that infusion of factor IX may result in anaphylaxis and nephrotic syndrome, limiting the ability to offer these patients ITI.[11]

FEIBA contains activated factor II, factor IX, factor X, and factor VII. Its mechanism of action is believed to be the promotion of thrombin formation on the platelet surface. Dosing is recommended at 50 to 100 IU/kg every 8 to 24 hours. It is recommended to not exceed 200 IU/kg per day to avoid thrombotic events.[11] Efficacy of FEIBA in controlling acute bleeding episodes has been reported to range from 80% to 100% and FEIBA is approximately 90% effective in controlling bleeding in surgical patients.[11] FEIBA may contain traces of factor VIII, however, and owing to the risk of anamnesis, some recommend against using FEIBA in patients who are planned to undergo ITI. Although there is a risk of thrombosis development with the use of FEIBA, this risk is exceedingly low, with 1 study demonstrating only 16 thrombotic events over a 10-year period of FEIBA use.[12]

rFVIIa bypasses the intrinsic coagulation pathway and enhances production of factor Xa on the platelet surface. This, in turn, leads to an increase in thrombin production, promoting platelet aggregation, activation of thrombin-activatable fibrinolysis inhibitor and factor XIII, and promotes the production of a fibrin plug. rFVIIIa has been used as a bypass agent in patients with inhibitors to treat acute bleeds as well as during surgical management. It is also used in a prophylactic manner and is used during ITI. rFVIIa has a short half-life (approximately 2.4 hours). During acute bleeding, rFVIIa may need to be administered every 2 to 3 hours until hemostasis is achieved.[8] During an acute bleed in a patient without inhibitors, 1 to 2 infusions of factor VIII will result in hemostasis in more than 90% of cases. In contrast, inhibitor patients with an acute bleed may require at least 3 or 4 infusions of rFVIIa to achieve hemostasis in 90% of cases. Administration of FEIBA every 12 hours results in control of approximately 76% of intraarticular bleeding after 36 hours.[9] When the efficacy of rFVIIa and FEIBA have been compared, some studies have suggested better efficacy in producing hemostasis with rFVIIa, whereas other studies have demonstrated equivalence. Some support preference for rFVIIa because of its decreased risk of causing an anamnestic response.[11] Serious thromboembolic events with administration of factor VIIa at a rate of less than 1%.[11]

ITI is highly encouraged in hemophilia A patients with inhibitors so that the patient can be administered factor VIII when necessary. ITI has been reported to eliminate inhibitors in approximately 80% of patients with hemophilia A with inhibitors and 30% of patients with hemophilia B with inhibitors.[9] It is especially beneficial to begin ITI in early childhood, because it may also prevent arthropathy.[7] If ITI is not successful, however, bleeding can only be managed with the administration of rFVIIa or FEIBA. There are a variety of ITI protocols that are used, but in general, the protocol consists of administration of repeated doses of factor VIII (sometimes twice per day). In addition, some protocols include immune suppression with the use of immunopheresis, cyclophosphamide, cyclosporine, mycophenolate mofetil, rituximab, or dexamethasone.[7,8] There are specific criteria that define success in ITI therapy. Part of the definition involves plasma factor VIII recovery. Testing factor VIII recovery involves measuring peak serum levels 30 minutes after factor VIII infusion and comparing this level with the expected increase in factor VIII based on the expectation that 1 U/kg of factor VIII should increase plasma factor VIII by 2%.[8] The consensus definition of success includes plasma factor VIII recovery of 66% or better than predicted, undetectable inhibitor level (<0.06 BU/mL), a factor VIII a half-life of 6 or more hours after a 72-hour factor VIII washout, and no anamnesis after additional factor VIII infusion. Definition of partial success entails plasma factor VIII recovery of less than 66% of predicted, inhibitor level less than 5 BU/mL, and a factor VIII half-life of less than 6 hours after a 72-hour factor VIII washout. Failure is defined as an inability to achieve complete or partial success within 33 months or less than 20% inhibitor titer reduction over a 6-month period after the first 3 months of ITI therapy.[8] The prognosis for success is considered good if the baseline inhibitor titer at the start of ITI is less than 10 BU/mL and peak titer has been less than 200 BU/mL.[8]

ACQUIRED HEMOPHILIA

Acquired hemophilia A (AHA) is a very rare, potentially fatal disorder that is reported to occur in 0.2 to 1.48 patients per million per year.[13] It is an autoimmune disorder marked by the development of autoantibodies (usually IgG), which inhibit factor VIII. It has a bimodal age distribution, with peaks in presentation in the ages of 20 to 40 and another peak in patients over the age of 60. More than 80% of patients are over the age of 65, with a median age of onset of 74 to 78 years. The younger patients tend to be females and presentation is often associated with pregnancy or collagen vascular disorders, with pregnancy accounting for approximately 2% to 15% of cases.[14] When occurring in association with pregnancy, it usually presents 1 to 4 months postpartum in a primipara. Pregnancy associated AHA typically carries a good prognosis because inhibitor titers tend to be relatively low (median of ~20 BU/mL) there is up to a 63% spontaneous remission rate after a mean of 30 months, and it carries a mortality rate reported in the range of 0% to 6%.[14] Besides pregnancy and collagen vascular disorders, other conditions associated with AHA may include malignancy, other auto-immune disorders, drug reactions (including beta-lactam antibiotics and nonsteroidal anti-inflammatory drugs, among others less commonly prescribed by oral surgeons), or dermatologic disease, but the most common cause is idiopathic.[14] Approximately 15% of AHA is associated with an autoimmune disorder. In contrast with pregnancy-associated AHA, these cases usually present with high titers and are unlikely to have spontaneous remission, usually requiring immunosuppressive treatment. Another 10% to 15% of cases are associated with malignancy. Management of the malignancy may result in eradication of the inhibitor, but failure to eradicate the inhibitor with treatment of the malignancy tends to be associated with a poor prognosis owing to advanced malignant disease.

AHA is a severe and often rapidly progressive bleeding disorder requiring hemostatic management and transfusion in 70% to 90% of patients with a mortality risk of 5% to 10% (besides the exception in pregnancy associated disease as described).[14] Subcutaneous, muscle, and mucosal bleeding are often reported. Intraarticular bleeding and bleeding in the central nervous system are rare. Approximately 5% to 10% of cases present postoperatively, so a patient with significant postoperative bleeding who falls into the aforementioned risk categories may possibly be presenting with AHA. Delays in diagnosis, which are common, may increase the likelihood of mortality. As in congenital hemophilia, AHA presents with an isolated elevation of PTT. A mixing study (described the congenital hemophilia section) will result in lack of correction of the PTT. If the mixing study suggests AHA, quantitative analysis of the inhibitor level is performed. Interestingly, inhibitors in AHA differ from inhibitors in congenital hemophilia in terms of factor VIII inactivation kinetics. In congenital hemophilia, the inhibitors exhibit "type 1" kinetics in that there is a linear relationship between the amount of inhibitor present and the residual factor VIII activity, with complete inactivation with high levels of inhibitors. In AHA, the inhibitors exhibit "type 2" kinetics, the inactivation pattern is not linear, and even high concentrations of inhibitor may not completely inactivate factor VIII activity. This complex kinetic order can lead to an inaccurate estimation of factor activity and can complicate management.[14]

Treatment is aimed at eradication of the inhibitor. If a patient with AHA requires a surgical procedure, it should be deferred if at all possible until the inhibitor is eradicated—even placement of an intravenous line can place the patient at risk of severe bleeding.[13,14] Acute management of the AHA patient involves management of bleeding as well as inhibitor eradication (immunosuppressive treatment). In acute bleeding, local hemostatic measures such as topical fibrin and antifibrinolytics should be used and FVIII bypassing agents, rFVIIa and FEIBA are recommended. Although there have not been comparative studies between the 2 in this setting, rFVIIa is the recommended first-line choice.[11] Appropriate duration of treatment is not known, but usually hemostasis is achieved within 24 to 72 hours. The combination of FEIBA and transexamic acid should be avoided owing to potential thromboembolic risk.[14] If bypassing agents are unavailable, plasma factor VIII concentrate (if titer is low and high doses of factor VIII can be administered) and desmopressin (DDAVP) with factor VIII (if the titer is low and the bleeding minor) may be administered. Severe hemorrhage in a high titer patient may also be managed via plasmapheresis or immunoadsorption. First-line therapy in inhibitor eradication (immunosuppressive treatment) includes prednisone with or without cyclophosphamide. Rituximab is considered a second-line alternative, with alternatives to Rituximab including cyclosporine, azathioprine, mycophenolate, and vincristine. High-dose immunoglobulin therapy is not recommended. It must be remembered that many of these patients are elderly, may be frail, and may be subject to increased risks of neutropenia, infection, or sepsis. Complete remission is reported in 70% to 80% of patients who receive corticosteroids with or without cyclophosphamide.[14] The median time to remission is 30 days. Inhibitor eradication is defined as undetectable inhibitor levels as well as a normal factor VIII level. Patients who have achieved successful remission are monitored with PTT and factor VIII level determinations every month for the first 6 months, then every 2 or 3 months for up to 1 year, and then every 6 months during the second year or longer.[14] Often, patients achieve high levels of factor VIII after remission and usually have comorbidities that predispose to thromboembolism, so these patients are recommended to have pharmacologic thromboprophylaxis, especially if they have high levels of factor VIII. Relapses do occur in approximately 15% to 24% of cases, with a median time to relapse of 3 to 4 months (7–9 months in some reports), although relapse can occur years later.[13,15]

MANAGEMENT OF HEMOPHILIA

Hemophiliac patients receive factor replacement in several scenarios: prophylactically, on-demand to treat bleeding episodes, or perioperatively. As mentioned, bleeding into joints repetitively results in hemarthroses, which ultimately can lead to a debilitating arthropathy. Hemophilic arthropathy is felt to be related to iron deposition in joints, leading to chronic inflammation and synovial hypertrophy and eventually cartilage destruction and subchondral bone damage occurs.[16] In regions where it is feasible economically, it is the standard of care to provide factor replacement in patients with severe Hemophilia A or B two or three times per week to prevent this complication.[2] In fact, this standard of care is recommended by the World Health Organization as well as the Medical and Scientific Advisory Council of the National Hemophilia Foundation USA.[16] Patients with mild or moderate hemophilia are managed in an on-demand manner, being administered factor replacement when a bleed occurs or surgery is planned.

For patients who are on hemophilia prophylaxis, it is clear that the earlier prophylaxis is begun, the better the success in reducing hemophilic arthropathy. It is essential that prophylaxis is begun before the occurrence of the first intraarticular bleed in severe hemophilia.[16,17] This is often around the age of 1.[18] In addition to the reduction in risk of arthropathy with early prophylaxis, the risk of life-threatening traumatic hemorrhage and intracranial hemorrhage are reduced. It is important to be aware that even high dose factor administration might not completely eliminate arthropathy in some patients.[18] Whether or not prophylaxis should be continued into adulthood is controversial.[16,17] Studies have shown that the number of bleeding events generally increases in young adults who switch from prophylaxis to on-demand treatment. Patients who tolerate this switch better tend to be patients who have milder bleeding issues.[17] Some recommend that prophylaxis continue at least until physical maturity has been reached and be reinstituted if significant hemarthroses recur.[16] A recent review of the literature indicated that approximately 45% of adults with hemophilia A included in the studies reviewed receive prophylaxis.[16] Another literature review by Oldenburg and Brackmann[16] indicated that approximately 27.3% of severe hemophiliac adolescents and adults can be withdrawn successfully from prophylaxis over a mean observation period of up to 19 years.

Reduction of hemophilic arthropathy is not the only benefit of prophylaxis. Patients who have been managed with prophylaxis rather than with on-demand treatment have a lower risk of inhibitor development.[18] Some patients, however, will likely have high-risk genetic mutations and will still form inhibitors despite prophylaxis.[17] Because patients with hemophilia B are at lower risk of developing inhibitors, a goal of prophylaxis in hemophilia B should only be to reduce arthropathy rather than reduce inhibitor development.

SURGICAL MANAGEMENT OF THE PATIENT WITH HEMOPHILIA

Surgical management of the hemophilia patient requires knowledge of the patient's level of severity, presence and responsiveness of inhibitors, and the history of how surgery has been managed in the past and the success of postoperative hemostasis. The appropriate management of these patients requires close consultation with the patient's hematologist and usually the patient and their family member will be able to provide a significant amount of helpful historical information concerning their disease state. In general, the goal is to raise factor (VIII or IX) concentrations to 80% to 100% just before surgery and a level of at least 50% should be maintained 5 to 14 days postoperatively.[1,2] For dental extractions, slightly less aggressive correction has been supported, with recommendations to achieve factor levels of 50% to 70% preoperatively and maintained at 50% for 5 to 7 days postoperatively.[19] Some have even suggested that 30% factor activity is sufficient.[19] Factors VIII and IX have short half-lives, with reports varying a little, but in general, factor VIII has a half-life of 6 to 16 hours and factor IX has a half-life ranging from 14 to 27 hours.[2,17] It has been noted that younger children tend to have shorter factor half-lives and may need more frequent factor dosing.[19] Long-acting factor formulations, many of which are pegylated forms, are in development and trial use. Long-acting factor has different peak and trough kinetics than traditional formulations, which will need to be taken into consideration with use, but pegylation does seem to increase the half-life of factor VIII approximately 1.5-fold and of factor IX by approximately 4- to 5-fold.[17]

Guidelines for factor replacement indicate that generally, 1.0 IU/kg of factor VIII is expected to increase the factor VIII level by 0.02 IU/mL, or 2%. Administration of 1.0 IU/kg of factor IX is expected to increase factor IX levels by 0.01 IU/ml or 1%.[2] This generally equates to a dose of 50 IU/kg of factor VIII concentrate or 100 IU/kg of factor IX concentrate in preparation for major surgery or to manage acute bleeding in a severe hemophiliac.[1,2] Factor should be administered within a 10- to 20-minute window before the procedure, because earlier infusion may result in decreasing levels by the time surgery begins.[20] It is useful to perform an assessment of plasma factor level just before surgery as well. Owing to the short half-lives, maintenance doses of factor VIII are usually administered every 12 hours in hemophilia A and of factor IX every 24 hours in hemophilia B.[1] Due to the high number of hemophilia A patients that develop inhibitors over their lifetime, it is advisable that inhibitor screening is performed within 1 week before planned surgery to ensure the planned factor VIII infusion will be effective.[20] Depending on the extensiveness of the surgery and its bleeding risk, it may be necessary to have factor concentrates available intraoperatively.

Some patients with mild or moderate hemophilia A may be managed perioperatively (in preparation for surgery or in response to acute bleeding) with administration of DDAVP via either intranasal, subcutaneous, or intravenous routes. In these patients, DDAVP may be expected to increase levels of factor VIII by 2- to 3-fold with a peak effect 30 to 60 minutes after administration. The half-life of released factor VIII is 8 to 12 hours, similar to native factor.[1,20] The recommended subcutaneous or intravenous dose is 0.3 µg/kg. It may need to be dosed every 12 hours, but in many cases, once daily dosing is sufficient. It is important to understand that not all patients respond to this regimen and it is important to determine the effect of DDAVP on factor levels before depending on this regimen perioperatively. It is also important to recognize that with repeated administration of DDAVP over a short period of time, tachyphylaxis may occur, resulting in decreasing factor level responsiveness. Additionally, because DDAVP is a synthetic analog of vasopressin, it can have the same effect as vasopressin, causing water reabsorption in the renal collecting ducts. Therefore, excessive water intake while DDAVP is being used should be avoided to decrease the likelihood of hyponatremia.[1]

As discussed, patients with low inhibitor titers who are low responders may be managed with simply higher doses of factor VIII or IX. However, in patients with high titer inhibitors who are high responders, either FEIBA or rFVIIa will be necessary. It is important to know that the hemostatic response to bypass agents is typically not as effective as with infusion of factor VIII or factor IX; therefore, there may be an increased risk of perioperative bleeding.[20] Various dosing recommendations are available. One of the recommendations includes a preoperative bolus of rFVIIa of 90 to 120 µg/kg. Subsequent doses recommended are 90 µg/kg every 2 hours for the first 48 hours, then 90 µg/kg every 3, 4, then 6 hours on days 3, 5, and 8 respectively. The recommended preoperative bolus of FEIBA is 75 to 100 IU/kg. Subsequent doses recommended are 70 IU/kg every 8 hours for a minimum of 3 days to a maximum of 200 IU/kg per day. Doses may be tapered starting on day 4 to 50 IU/kg every 8 hours.[20]

Several adjuncts are available to assist with hemostasis during oral surgery procedures. Certainly, one may wish to use absorbable gelatin sponges, collagen plugs, absorbable fibrillary hemostatic agents, topical thrombin, and sutures at the surgical site to directly enhance hemostasis. Antifibrinolytics such as transexamic acid or epsilon-aminocaproic acid are recommended additions to increase the efficacy of hemostasis. Antifibrinolytics competitively inhibit plasminogen and decrease clot breakdown. Both transexamic acid and epsilon-aminocaproic acid can be used topically via soaked gauze for the patient to bite down on, as well as systemically. Ideally, the antifibrinolytic should be started before the surgery and continued for 7 days postoperatively.[19]

Procedures that may cause bleeding, especially in areas adjacent to the airway where compression cannot be applied, should be avoided. It is best if one can avoid administering an inferior alveolar nerve block; in some patients, buccal infiltration using 4% articaine with 1:100,000 epinephrine may provide sufficient anesthesia to mandibular posterior teeth. Floor of the mouth injections should be strictly avoided. After dental extractions in a hemophiliac, the patient should be instructed to bite down on gauze for longer than the average patient—at least 1 hour and maybe 2 hours. Consideration should be given to keeping the patient in the office longer to observe for hemostasis; depending on the circumstances, this may be for up to 2 hours. Additionally, medications that may cause bleeding such as aspirin and nonsteroidal antiinflammatories should not be recommended or prescribed. Hemophiliac patients should be followed closely postoperatively to ensure continued hemostasis and additionally, management of an enlarged "liver clot" may be necessary. A "liver clot" may result from continued disruption of the clotting process with additional bleeding with some incomplete clotting occurring in a repeated manner. A patient who presents with this complication will need additional factor infusion and a procedure completed to clean out the clot and any material/foreign bodies that may be contributing to its formation, and achievement of good hemostasis with suture, topical agents, and pressure. Surgeries should be performed early in the week to facilitate in-office follow-up appointments in the office. This author's preference is to perform surgery on a Monday and have the patient return for follow-up appointments on Wednesday and Friday.

In general, hemophiliacs are believed to be at low risk for thromboembolism. However, the administration of factor concentrates can increase the risk of thromboembolism, especially in patients who are undergoing procedures with increased thromboembolic risk, such as orthopedic procedures or procedures that will result in decreased mobility. Other risk factors include use of long-term central venous access, and the use of bypassing agents or intensive factor replacement therapy.[21] The administration of FEIBA has been reported with a thromboembolic risk of 4 to 8.4 per 100,000 infusions, whereas the risk of thromboembolism with infusion of rFVIIa is significantly lower.[21] In most patients who are at risk, compression stockings, sequential compression devices, and early mobilization should be sufficient to prevent venous thromboembolism. Factors that may increase the risk of thromboembolism may include age greater than 60 years, obesity, personal or family history of venous thromboembolism, and confirmed thrombophilia. There is no established recommendation for thromboprophylaxis in hemophilia patients who are at a higher level of risk, but the following have been reported: low molecular weight heparin, unfractionated heparin, warfarin, or fondaparinux.[21]

SUMMARY

Hemophilia will be encountered in the oral surgeon's office. Appropriate management of these patients requires a thorough understanding of the levels of severity of the disease in addition to an understanding of the effect of inhibitors. Thoughtful coordination with the patient's hematologist is required before any procedure, as either infusion of factor, DDAVP, or bypassing agents may be required. Surgical management of these patients not only requires adequate preparation but also close follow-up to evaluate for postoperative bleeding complications.

REFERENCES

1. Zimmerman B, Valentino LA. Hemophilia: in review. Pediatr Rev 2013;34(7):289–95.
2. Fijnvandraat K, Cnossen MH, Leebeek FW, et al. Diagnosis and management of hemophilia. BMJ 2012;344:1–5.
3. Pavlova A, Oldenburg J. Defining severity of hemophilia: more than factor levels. Semin Thromb Hemost 2013;39:702–10.
4. Schramm W. The history of hemophilia—a short review. Thromb Res 2014;134:S4–9.
5. Franchini M. The modern treatment of hemophilia: a narrative review. Blood Transfus 2013;11:178–82.
6. Lippi G, Franchini M, Montagnana M, et al. Inherited disorders of blood coagulation. Ann Med 2012;44: 405–18.
7. Kreuz W, Ettingshausen CE. Inhibitors in patients with haemophilia A. Thromb Res 2014;134:S22–6.
8. DeFrates SR, McDonagh KT, Adams VR. The reversal of inhibitors in congenital hemophilia. Pharmacotherapy 2013;33(2):157–64.
9. Gomez K, Klamroth R, Mahlangu J, et al. Key issues in inhibitor management in patients with haemophilia. Blood Transfus 2014;12(Suppl 1):s319–29.
10. Peyvandi F, Mannucci PM, Gargiola I, et al. 5 source of factor VIII replacement (plasmatic or recombinant) and incidence of inhibitory alloantibodies in previously untreated patients with severe hemophilia A: The Multicenter Randomized Sippet Study. American Society of Hematology 57th Annual Meeting and Exposition. Orlando (FL), December 6, 2015.
11. Franchini M, Coppola A, Tagliaferri A, et al. FEIBA versus novoseven in hemophilia patients with inhibitors. Semin Thromb Hemost 2013;39:772–8.
12. Ehrlich HJ, Henzl MJ, Gomperts ED, et al. Safety of factor VIII inhibitor bypass activity (FEIBA): 10-year compilation of thrombotic adverse events. Haemophilia 2002;8(2):83–90.
13. Webert K. Acquired hemophilia A. Semin Thromb Hemost 2012;38:735–41.
14. Coppola A, Favaloro EJ, Tufano A, et al. Acquired inhibitors of coagulation factors: part I—acquired hemophilia A. Semin Thromb Hemost 2012;38:433–46.
15. Sborov DW, Rodgers GM. How I manage patients with acquired hemophilia A. Br J Haematol 2013; 161:157–65.
16. Oldenburg J, Brackmann HH. Prophylaxis in adult patients with severe hemophilia A. Thromb Res 2014;134:S33–7.
17. Ljung R, Andersson NG. The current status of prophylactic replacement therapy in children and adults with haemophilia. Br J Haematol 2015;169: 777–86.
18. Schwarz R, Ljung R, Tedgård U. Various regimens for prophylactic treatment of patients with haemophilia. Eur J Haematol 2015;94(Suppl 77):11–6.
19. Ljung R, Knobe K. How to manage invasive procedures in children with haemophilia. Br J Haematol 2012;157:519–28.
20. Mensah PK, Gooding R. Surgery in patients with inherited bleeding disorders. Anaesthesia 2015; 70(Suppl 1):112–20.
21. Ozelo MC. Surgery in patients with hemophilia: is thromboprophylaxis mandatory? Thromb Res 2012; 130:S23–6.

Hypercoagulable States
What the Oral Surgeon Needs to Know

Robert Bona, MD*

KEYWORDS

- Thrombophilia • Hypercoagulable • Factor V Leiden • Protein C • Protein S

KEY POINTS

- Factor V Leiden and prothrombin G20210A gene mutations are relatively common inherited thrombophilic abnormalities in the Caucasian population conferring the individual with a small increase risk for venous thrombosis.
- Antithrombin, protein C, and protein S deficiency are less common abnormalities that confer the individual with a significantly higher risk for venous thrombosis.
- The development of phospholipid antibodies is an autoimmune condition that predisposes the individual to arterial thrombosis, venous thrombosis, and/or pregnancy loss.
- Cancer is a common cause of thrombophilia.
- Long-term anticoagulation is often considered in these individuals; but treatment should be individualized, balancing the risk of thrombosis with the risk of bleeding with anticoagulant drugs.

NORMAL HEMOSTASIS

Normal clotting of the blood relies on several component parts, including functional platelets, intact endothelium, and normal coagulation proteins to name the most obvious elements. Physiologic clot formation in response to injury is limited by several anticoagulant proteins/factors. In the same way, abnormal clotting (thrombosis) is also prevented by the presence of these same factors. Although a deficiency of a procoagulant clotting protein (factor VIII) can lead to a bleeding disorder, a deficiency of or abnormality of these anticoagulant factors can lead to a hypercoagulable or thrombophilic condition.[1,2]

MAJOR ANTICOAGULANT MECHANISMS OF BLOOD
Endothelial Cell

The endothelium serves several important functions in the prevention of clot extension outside the direct area of injury and prevention of thrombosis.[3]

- First and foremost, the endothelial cells serve as a barrier between the flowing blood and the underlying stroma (collagen) and cells. Collagen is able to engage von Willebrand factor in the blood and begin the process of platelet adhesion, and subendothelial cells (smooth muscle cells, pericytes, fibroblasts) express tissue factor on their surface. Tissue factor interaction with factor VIIa in the blood will result in the rapid initiation of the coagulation cascade and fibrin deposition.
- Secondly, the endothelium synthesizes and secretes products that impair platelet aggregation. These products include the arachidonic acid metabolite, prostacyclin (PGI_2), and CD39, which is an ADPase. This enzyme degrades ADP to AMP and then adenosine, thereby neutralizing the potent proaggregation effect of ADP on circulating platelets.

Disclosures: None.
Frank H. Netter School of Medicine, Quinnipiac University, 275 Mount Carmel Avenue, MNH 307L, Hamden, CT 06518-1908, USA
* Corresponding author. North Haven Campus, 370 Bassett Road, MNH 307L, North Haven, CT 06473
E-mail address: robert.bona@quinnipiac.edu

Oral Maxillofacial Surg Clin N Am 28 (2016) 491–495
http://dx.doi.org/10.1016/j.coms.2016.06.002
1042-3699/16/$ – see front matter © 2016 Elsevier Inc. All rights reserved.

- The production of glycosaminoglycans and expression of those compounds on the surface of endothelial cells: These complex proteoglycans enhance that action of anti-thrombin (AT) (see later discussion) as a potent inhibitor of the serine proteases in the coagulation reactions.
- Expression of thrombomodulin and the protein C (PC) receptor: The interaction of these receptors with their ligands results in the conversion of the zymogen PC to its active enzymatic form (activated PC) (see later discussion).
- Tissue factor pathway inhibitor (TFPI): TFPI is an inhibitor of the tissue factor pathway of coagulation. It initially binds to activated factor X (Xa) and the complex binds to the tissue factor-VII complex, thereby inhibiting the activity of the tissue factor.
- Fibrinolytic proteins: The endothelium can synthesize and secrete both profibrinolytic and antifibrinolytic proteins (tissue plasminogen activator and plasminogen activator inhibitor, respectively).

Circulating Proteins

Antithrombin

AT (previously known as AT-III) is a member of the serine protease inhibitor family of proteins. It is synthesized in the liver and circulates in the blood. It has a reactive center that interacts with active serine residue of the coagulation protein (serine enzyme). Once the enzyme cleaves the reactive center, a complex is formed (AT plus coagulation enzyme), which is cleared from the circulation (**Fig. 1**). Heparin binding to AT increases the availability of the reactive site allowing for a significantly enhanced activity. The endothelial cell–expressed glycosaminoglycans act in this fashion. The serine proteases that are inactivated in this way are primarily IIa (thrombin), factor Xa, and factor IXa.

Protein C/Protein S

PC and protein S (PS) are both vitamin K–dependent proteins synthesized by the liver and post-translationally modified by the carboxylation of the gamma carbon on the glutamic acid residues on the amino acid terminus of the proteins. PC is a zymogen and requires activation to its active form by limited proteolysis. This activation occurs by the enzyme thrombin, which is brought into close proximity to the necessary cleavage site on PC by binding to the endothelial receptor, thrombomodulin.[4] The activation of PC is optimized by the precise expression of thrombomodulin and the endothelial cell PC receptor (EPCR). When thrombin binds to thrombomodulin and PC binds to its receptor (EPCR), the bound thrombin is able to catalyze the conversion of PC to activated PC (APC). APC along with its cofactor, PS, is able to proteolyze and inactivate coagulation factors Va and VIIIa (**Fig. 2**). This inactivation occurs optimally on endothelial cell surfaces. Notably, PS exists in 2 forms in the blood, approximately 40% free in the circulation and approximately 60% bound to the complement binding protein, C4b-binding protein. It is only the free PS that can serve as the cofactor for APC activity.

HYPERCOAGULABLE CONDITIONS (SELECTED)

- Inherited
  - AT deficiency
  - PC deficiency

Antithrombin (III)

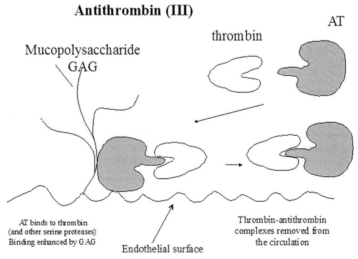

Mucopolysaccharide GAG

thrombin

AT

AT binds to thrombin
(and other serine proteases)
Binding enhanced by GAG

Endothelial surface

Thrombin-antithrombin
complexes removed from
the circulation

Fig. 1. Mechanism of action of AT. GAG, glycosaminoglycan.

Protein C/Protein S

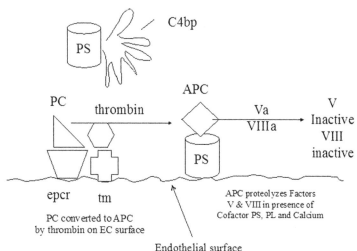

Fig. 2. Mechanism of action of PC and PS. EC, endothelial cell.

- ○ PS deficiency
- ○ Factor V Leiden
- ○ Prothrombin gene mutation (G20210A)
- ○ Homocysteinemia
- • Acquired
  - ○ Cancer
  - ○ Myeloproliferative disorders (polycythemia vera, essential thrombocytosis)
  - ○ Phospholipid antibodies
  - ○ Hormone
    - ■ Pregnancy
    - ■ Post partum
    - ■ Oral contraceptive use
    - ■ Hormone replacement therapy
  - ○ Medications
    - ■ Thalidomide/lenalidomide/ pomalidomide
    - ■ Bevacizumab
    - ■ Tamoxifen
  - ○ Immobility
  - ○ Major surgery
  - ○ Acquired deficiencies of AT, PC, or PS
  - ○ Human immunodeficiency virus/AIDS

AT deficiency[5] is an unusual condition resulting from either a deficiency of or alteration in the function of AT. When inherited, this is an autosomal dominant disorder. Acquired conditions can be seen with nephrotic syndrome. Patients are primarily at risk for venous thromboembolism. Interestingly, patients on anticoagulant therapy with heparin (including low-molecular-weight heparin) may not have an adequate plasma response because these drugs work through their binding to AT.

PC deficiency[6] is an unusual condition resulting from either a deficiency of or an alteration in the function of PC. It is an autosomal dominant disorder, and individuals with homozygous abnormalities present with diffuse thrombosis and hemorrhage (into infarcted tissue) early in the postnatal period. This condition, purpura fulminans,[7] is life threatening and requires therapy with PC concentrates. Warfarin-induced skin necrosis may also be seen in individuals with PC deficiency. Because PC is a vitamin K–dependent protein, its levels will decrease with the use of warfarin. The half-life of PC is relatively short (6–8 hours), so PC levels may decrease quicker than the coagulation proteins (prothrombin and factors VII, IX, and X) in the initial stages of warfarin use. This decrease is most often seen with large loading doses of warfarin, which should be avoided.

PS deficiency[8] is characterized by many of the same clinical associations as PC deficiency. PS deficiency may be caused by a low protein level, abnormally functioning protein, or by a low free but normal total PS.

Functional assays are more useful in the diagnosis of AT, PC, or PS deficiency than antigenic assays. AT, PC, and PS deficiency have relatively high relative risks for venous thromboembolism.

Factor V Leiden[9] is a relatively common abnormality, especially in Caucasian individuals whereby it is estimated that between 5% and 7% of the population has this change in the factor V DNA/protein structure rendering the molecule partially resistant to inactivation by APC. Twenty percent to 30% of individuals with hereditary thrombophilia and thrombosis will have factor V Leiden. It is an autosomal dominant disorder, with individuals with homozygous mutations having a very high risk of venous thrombosis.

Prothrombin G20201A gene mutation[10] results from a mutation in the coding sequence of the prothrombin gene (guanine exchanged for by adenine at nucleic acid position 20210). This mutation causes approximately 30% more prothrombin being synthesized (circulating plasma results approximately 130% of normal), which places individuals at risk for venous thrombosis. This is also inherited in an autosomal dominant fashion.

See **Box 1** for a summary of common features among the aforementioned hypercoagulable conditions.

Homocysteinemia is an uncommon condition that predisposes individuals to both arterial and venous thromboembolism. It had been previously thought that individuals with mild elevations of serum homocysteine or individuals with a mutation in the 5′ methylene tetrahydrofolate reductase enzyme were at risk for thromboembolism, but this is no longer thought to be the case.

Cancer is a clear risk factor for the development of venous thrombosis. Trousseau syndrome is widely used to describe the individual with cancer who has had a thrombotic event. The precise description refers to migratory superficial thrombophlebitis in people with cancer. Although most individuals with cancer who develop thrombosis have the diagnosis of cancer firmly established, it is well known that some individuals may develop a venous thromboembolic event many months before the diagnosis of cancer is made.[11] This phenomenon probably represents a hypercoagulable state existing in the setting of clinically occult cancer yet to be recognized. The mechanism for the association between thrombosis and cancer relates to increase tissue factor production by cancer cells or tumor-associated macrophages as well as other procoagulants produced by the cancer cells.

Phospholipid antibodies are a complex set of antibodies that put patients at risk for venous thrombosis, arterial thrombosis, and premature pregnancy loss.[12] These antibodies have been variably known as lupus anticoagulants, anticardiolipin antibodies, and phospholipid antibodies adding to the confusion around their understanding. These heterogeneous antibodies recognize protein phospholipid complexes that interfere with anticoagulant function of the blood or the endothelium. Major antigens recognized by these antibodies include B_2 glycoprotein I, cardiolipin, PC, prothrombin, annexins, and others.[13] Because of the phospholipid-binding properties of these antibodies, they cause the common coagulation test, activated partial thromboplastin time (APTT), to be prolonged, an association usually associated with a bleeding disorder. However, in this condition, the predisposition toward thrombosis is due to the antibodies interaction with the aforementioned named proteins (and others). It is generally agreed on that individuals who have developed thrombosis in association with phospholipid antibodies are at significant risk for recurrent thrombosis if not treated with long-term anticoagulation (**Box 2**).

Medications, including thalidomide and its analogues (lenalidomide and pomalidomide) used to treat multiple myeloma, tamoxifen used primarily for the treatment of estrogen receptor–positive breast cancer, and bevacizumab (a monoclonal antibody directed against vascular endothelial growth factor) used to most often to treat colorectal cancer, have been associated with an increased risk for thrombosis.

DIAGNOSIS OF INHERITED HYPERCOAGULABLE CONDITIONS

- Plasma *functional* assays for AT, PC, and PS are most useful and will capture patients who have an abnormality in protein function but normal protein levels.[14]
- Pitfalls in the diagnosis of AT, PC, and PS deficiency include
  - Levels may be altered in individuals on anticoagulant therapy
  - Levels may be altered during normal pregnancy
  - Specialized laboratory testing usually required

Box 1
Common features of antithrombin, protein C, protein S deficiency, factor V Leiden, and prothrombin gene mutation include

- Autosomal dominant disorders
- Increased risk for *venous* thrombosis
- Thrombosis at a young age
- Thrombosis at unusual sites (portal vein, retinal v)

Box 2
Salient features of phospholipid antibodies

- Increase risk for venous and arterial thrombosis and pregnancy loss
- Significant risk for recurrent thrombosis if not treated with anticoagulant drugs
- Often prolong the APTT

- Factor V Leiden and prothrombin gene mutation assays are done with polymerase chain reaction technology and are highly reliable and not altered by medication use or the clinical situation of the individual.

TREATMENT OF HYPERCOAGULABLE CONDITIONS

Treatment decisions usually depend on the severity of the hypercoagulable condition (eg, factor V Leiden vs AT deficiency), history and circumstance of thrombosis, bleeding risk for anticoagulant drugs, patient preferences, and other variables. These decisions are often complex, and an individualized approach is often used based on published high-quality evidence when available. Multiple anticoagulant drugs are available for use. By far the most commonly used drug has been warfarin, but parenteral heparin (in particular low-molecular-weight heparin) and so-called novel oral anticoagulants are in use as well. Discontinuation of anticoagulant drugs in these individuals in preparation for oral surgery should best be done in consultation with the patients' physician, in particular, that individual who is responsible for monitoring the anticoagulation therapy. Sometimes physician specialist input (vascular surgeon, hematologist, pulmonary physician) may also be required.

REFERENCES

1. Adams RL, Bird RJ. Review article: coagulation cascade and therapeutics update: relevance to nephrology. Part 1: overview of coagulation, thrombophilias and history of anticoagulants. Nephrology (Carlton) 2009;14:462–70.
2. Esmon C. Basic mechanisms and pathogenesis of venous thrombosis. Blood Rev 2009;23(5):225–9.
3. Pober J, Wang M, Bradley J. Mechanisms of endothelial dysfunction, injury, and death. Annu Rev Pathol 2009;4:71–95.
4. Anastasiou G, Gialeraki A, Merkouri E, et al. Thrombomodulin as a regulator of the anticoagulant pathway: implication in the development of thrombosis. Blood Coagul Fibrinolysis 2012;23:1–10.
5. Patnaik M, Moll S. Inherited antithrombin deficiency: a review. Haemophilia 2008;14:1229–39.
6. Bovill E, Bauer K, Dickerman J, et al. The clinical spectrum of heterozygous protein C deficiency in a large New England kindred. Blood 1989;73:712–7.
7. Dreyfus M, Magny J, Bridey F. Treatment of homozygous protein C deficiency and neonatal purpura fulminans with a purified protein C concentrate. N Engl J Med 1991;325:1564–8.
8. Ten Kate M, Van Der Meer J. Protein S deficiency: a clinical perspective. Haemophilia 2008;14:1222–8.
9. Kujovich J. Factor V Leiden thrombophilia. Genet Med 2011;13(1):1–16.
10. De Stefano V, Martinelli I, Mannucci P, et al. The risk of recurrent venous thromboembolism among heterozygous carriers of the G20210 prothrombin gene mutation. Br J Haematol 2001;113(3):630–5.
11. Sorensen H, Mellemkjaer L, Steffensen F, et al. The Risk of a diagnosis of cancer after primary deep venous thrombosis or pulmonary embolism. N Engl J Med 1998;338:1169–73.
12. Levin J, Branch D, Rauch J. The antiphospholipid syndrome. N Engl J Med 2002;346:752–63.
13. Giannakopoulos B, Krillis S. The pathogenesis of the antiphospholipid syndrome. N Engl J Med 2013;368:1033–44.
14. Moll S. Thrombophilias—practical implications and testing caveats. J Thromb Thrombolysis 2006;21(1):7–15.

Aspirin, Plavix, and Other Antiplatelet Medications
What the Oral and Maxillofacial Surgeon Needs to Know

Andre E. Ghantous, MD[a],
Elie M. Ferneini, DMD, MD, MHS, MBA[b,c,d],*

KEYWORDS

- Antiplatelet therapy • Aspirin • Bleeding • Myocardial infarction • Clopidogrel
- Coronary artery disease • Cardiac stenting • Angioplasty

KEY POINTS

- Most patients with coronary artery disease and peripheral vascular disease are on long-term antiplatelet therapy and dual therapy.
- Achieving a balance between ischemic and bleeding risk remains a challenge in patients undergoing surgery who are treated with dual antiplatelet therapy.
- For most outpatient oral and maxillofacial surgical procedures, maintenance and continuation of the antiplatelet therapy are recommended.

INTRODUCTION

Long-term antiplatelet therapy is an important component of secondary prevention after a cerebrovascular accident (CVA), transient ischemic attack, myocardial infarction (MI), or myocardial revascularization, or for patients with a diagnosis of peripheral arterial disease (PAD) or acute coronary syndrome (ACS). In fact, dual-antiplatelet therapy (eg, aspirin and clopidogrel) is commonly used in surgical patients. This therapy prevents stent thrombosis following percutaneous coronary intervention with placement of bare-metal or drug-eluting stents. In the perioperative period, the indication for antiplatelet agents is reinforced by the increased platelet activity following surgery; however, they also increase the risk of perioperative as well as postoperative surgical bleeding. The oral and maxillofacial surgeon must decide whether the risk of hemorrhage with antiplatelet therapy is lower than the risk of thrombosis when antiplatelet agents are stopped or disrupted.

Antiplatelet agents are categorized according to their mechanism of action: thromboxane/cyclooxygenase (COX) inhibitors, adenosine diphosphate receptor inhibitors, phosphodiesterase inhibitors, adenosine reuptake inhibitors, and glycoprotein IIb/IIIa inhibitors (**Fig. 1**).

THROMBOXANE/CYCLOOXYGENASE INHIBITOR
Aspirin (Acetylsalicylic Acid)

In 1763, Hippocrates prescribed willow tree bark extract for headaches.[1] Salicylic acid, the active ingredient of aspirin, was isolated from the bark

[a] Division of Cardiology, Department of Medicine, Yale University School of Medicine, 333 Cedar St., New Haven, CT 06510, USA; [b] Private Practice, Greater Waterbury OMS, 435 Highland Avenue, Suite 100, Cheshire, CT 06410, USA; [c] Beau Visage Med Spa, 435 Highland Avenue, Suite 100, Cheshire, CT 06410, USA; [d] Division of Oral and Maxillofacial Surgery, Department of Craniofacial Sciences, University of Connecticut, 263 Farmington Avenue, Farmington, CT 06030, USA.
* Corresponding author. Beau Visage Med Spa, 435 Highland Avenue, Suite 100, Cheshire, CT 06410, USA.
E-mail address: eferneini@yahoo.com

Oral Maxillofacial Surg Clin N Am 28 (2016) 497–506
http://dx.doi.org/10.1016/j.coms.2016.06.003

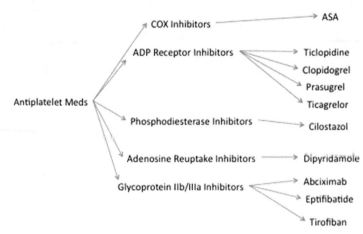

Fig. 1. Antiplatelet agents.

of the willow tree by Edward Stone of Wadham College.[2] Felix Hoffmann, from Bayer, was credited with the synthesis of aspirin in 1897, which is a registered trademark by Bayer with the generic term of acetylsalicylic acid (ASA).[3] John Robert Vane was actually awarded the Noble Prize in 1971 for showing how ASA suppresses the production of prostaglandins and thromboxane.

Low-dose ASA (40–100 mg) irreversibly blocks thromboxane A2 in platelets, leading to an inhibitory effect on platelet aggregation during the life of the affected platelets. This antithrombotic property makes ASA useful for reducing cardiovascular as well as thrombotic events. In addition, ASA is nonselective and irreversibly inhibits both forms of cyclooxygenase isozymes (COX-1 and COX-2). Higher doses of ASA will also inhibit prostaglandin A2 synthesis. The most common side effect of ASA is bleeding, especially if associated with another antiplatelet or anticoagulant agent. Patients who use immediate-release ASA (not enteric coated) and take a single dose of ibuprofen 400 mg should dose the ibuprofen at least 30 minutes or longer after ASA ingestion, or more than 8 hours before ASA ingestion in order to avoid attenuation of ASA's effect.

ASA has been shown to reduce cardiovascular events (MI, CVA, and death) in patients with high cardiovascular risk factors as well as decrease the risk of colorectal and endometrial cancer.[4–6] ASA therapy has net benefits in the acute phase of an evolving MI and should be administered to all patients with an evolving acute MI. In fact, ASA therapy has statistically significant reductions in the risk of vascular mortality (23%), nonfatal reinfarction (49%), and nonfatal stroke (46%). To achieve an immediate clinical antithrombotic effect, an initial minimum loading dose of 162 mg of ASA should be used in an acute MI.[7] In addition,

long-term ASA therapy has benefits on risk reduction of subsequent MI, stroke, and vascular death among patients with a wide range of prior manifestations of cardiovascular disease. The most widely tested regimen was a medium dose of ASA (75–325 mg/d). Most studies have shown no evidence that higher doses of ASA are more effective than daily ASA in this dose range.[8]

ADENOSINE DIPHOSPHATE RECEPTOR INHIBITORS

1. Thienopyridine class
   a. Ticlopidine (Ticlid)
   b. Clopidogrel (Plavix)
   c. Prasugrel (Effient)
2. Cyclopentyltriazolopyrimidine (CPTP)
   a. Ticagrelor (Brilinta)

Ticlopidine (Ticlid)

Ticlid, a thienopyridine, is an adenosine diphosphate (ADP) receptor inhibitor discovered in the 1970s and approved in 1978 in Europe for CVA therapy for patients who could not tolerate ASA. Thirteen years later, it was approved in the United States as a stronger antiplatelet agent than ASA to prevent coronary stent thrombosis when taken with ASA.[9] In addition to bleeding, ticlopidine has a serious adverse event, thrombotic thrombocytopenic purpura (TTP). After the approval of clopidogrel in 1997, which is less likely to cause TTP, the use of ticlopidine started declining, and as of April 2015, ticlopidine is no longer available on the US market.[10]

Clopidogrel (Plavix)

Clopidogrel is an oral thienopyridine antiplatelet that irreversibly inhibits the P2Y12 receptor on the ADP chemoreceptor of the platelet cellular membrane. The dosage is 75 mg once daily after a bolus dose of 300/600 mg and is approved for the treatment of ACS, which includes ST elevation MI, non-ST elevation MI, or unstable angina, in addition to ASA.[9–12] It is also approved for chronic therapy for stable ischemic heart disease, ischemic stroke, and peripheral vascular disease (PVD).[13–18] The most common adverse event is bleeding, which is increased when associated with ASA or anticoagulants. In addition, TTP is one of the rare adverse events but is much less frequent than with ticlopidine (4/1,000,000 patients).

Clopidogrel is a prodrug that requires activation in the liver by CYP2C19 and irreversibly inhibits the P2Y12 subtype of the ADP receptor. Patients who have a variant allele of CYP2C19 may be resistant to clopidogrel and have higher cardiovascular events if treated with clopidogrel in a setting of ACS.

Prasugrel (Effient)

Prasugrel is a thienopyridine class of ADP receptor inhibitors, like ticlopidine and clopidogrel. It irreversibly binds to the P2Y12 receptors. It is a prodrug and is actually more rapidly absorbed than clopidogrel and reduces platelet aggregation more potently and rapidly than clopidogrel. Its function is not affected by CYP2C19 liver enzyme and is not affected by coadministration of proton pump inhibitors (PPIs). It is approved for patients presenting with ACS with a percutaneous coronary intervention strategy.[19] The main side effects have been bleeding, and to a rare extent, TTP. Prasugrel's loading dose is 60 mg followed by 10 mg once daily, or 5 mg daily if the patient weighs less than 60 kg or is older than 75 years of age. Prasugrel has been shown to be superior to clopidogrel in reducing cardiovascular events with a slight increased risk of bleeding.

Ticagrelor (Brilinta)

Ticagrelor is a CPTP, like thienopyridine. Its mechanism of action is to block ADP receptors of P2Y12 subtype. In contrast to the other antiplatelet drugs, ticagrelor has a binding site different from ADP, making it an allosteric antagonist, and its blockage is reversible.

Ticagrelor is an active drug and does not need hepatic activation like the other thienopyridines. The variant allele of CYP2C19 has no effect on its efficacy. The US Food and Drug Administration (FDA) approved ticagrelor in July 2011 as a dual antiplatelet therapy for patients presenting with ACS for medical therapy or invasive therapeutic strategy. It has been shown to be superior to clopidogrel for reducing cardiovascular death, MI, and stroke with slightly more bleeding complications. In 2015, the FDA expanded the indication of ticagrelor to include patients with ischemic heart disease after 12 months following an ACS.[20] The ACS dosage is 180 mg orally as a bolus dose followed by 90 mg twice daily and 60 mg twice daily for chronic ischemic heart disease.[21] Most common side effects are bleeding and dyspnea.

PHOSPHODIESTERASE INHIBITORS
Cilostazol (Pletal)

Cilostazol is a selective inhibitor of type 3 phosphodiesterase with a therapeutic focus on increasing cyclic adenosine monophosphate (cAMP), leading to platelet aggregation inhibition and vasodilatation. Cilostazol is approved for the treatment of intermittent claudication.[22] The dosage is 120 mg twice daily and should be avoided in patients with uncontrolled congestive heart failure. Grapefruit juice may increase the drug's maximum concentration by 50%.[23]

ADENOSINE REUPTAKE INHIBITORS
Dipyridamole (Persantine)

Dipyridamole inhibits phosphodiesterase enzyme, leading to higher cellular cAMP and blocking platelet aggregation. It also blocks cellular uptake of adenosine and increases extracellular concentration of adenosine, leading to vasodilatation.[14] It also inhibits proliferation of smooth muscle cells in vivo and increases patency of synthetic atrioventricular hemodialysis grafts.[24] It is approved in combination with ASA for secondary prevention of stroke without increasing the bleeding risk.[14] Intravenous dipyridamole infusion is approved for cardiac nuclear stress testing because of its vasodilatory effect. Caffeine and aminophylline reverse the dilatory effects of dipyridamole.

INTRAVENOUS ANTIPLATELETS
Glycoprotein IIb/IIIa Inhibitors

Glycoprotein IIb/IIIa inhibitors are antagonists that are approved for acute therapy for patients presenting with ACS in conjunction with intravenous (IV) anticoagulants.[25–27]

Abciximab (ReoPro)
Abciximab is a monoclonal antibody that irreversibly inhibits glycoprotein IIb/IIIa, leading to inhibition of platelet aggregation.[25] The most common side effect is a higher risk of bleeding and thrombocytopenia. Being a Fab fragment, the patient can develop specific antibodies that can lead to

decreased efficacy with repeated administration. Abciximab can be administered in patients with advanced renal failure.

Eptifibatide (Integrilin)

Eptifibatide is a cyclic heptapeptide that reversibly binds to glycoprotein IIb/IIIa, leading to inhibition of platelet aggregation.[26] It has a short half-life and is indicated for patients presenting with an ACS in conjunction with IV anticoagulant for medical and invasive therapy. It is renally excreted and should be avoided in patients with advanced and chronic renal failure. Side effects are mainly bleeding and thrombocytopenia.

Tirofiban (Aggrastat)

Tirofiban is a glycoprotein IIb/IIIa inhibitor approved for patients presenting with an ACS undergoing percutaneous intervention.[27] It binds reversibly to glycoprotein IIb/IIIa with a short half-life and in conjunction with IV anticoagulant. It is renally excreted, and the main side effects are bleeding and thrombocytopenia.

ANTIPLATELET THERAPY

Antiplatelet therapy is a mainstay in the management of patients with coronary artery disease (CAD) and PVD. ASA is effective in dosages ranging between 75 and 325 mg per day. As discussed earlier, clopidogrel (75 mg per day) is a prodrug oxidized by hepatic cytochromes into an active metabolite. Some lipophilic statins, PPIs, and midazolam compete with clopidogrel for the same cytochromes and may potentially reduce its level of active metabolite by up to 30%. After cessation of ASA or clopidogrel, platelet aggregation returns to baseline in 5 days. There are actually no major differences in bleeding risk between ASA and clopidogrel when administered alone. Compared with clopidogrel, Effient is more effective at preventing stent thrombosis, but it increases the bleeding risk by 30%. However, the incidence of serious bleeding is not increased.

Most patients with CAD and PAD are on dual antiplatelet therapy. In fact, this therapy is mandatory after an ACS, a stent implantation, and an MI. Coronary lesions and stents behave like unstable plaques as long as they are not fully covered by a cellular layer. Endothelialization varies between bare-metal and drug-eluting stents. In general, the metal frame of a bare-metal stent is covered by an acellular matrix secreted by smooth muscle cells within 2 to 4 weeks after implantation.[28] Drug-eluting stents have a much slower endothelialization rate: 13% at 3 months and 56% at 3 years.[29] Therefore, the recommended duration of ADP-receptor blockers treatment is 4 weeks after bare-metal stents and at least 12 months after drug-eluting stents (**Table 1**).[30–32] Some other factors have a high predictive value for thrombotic events. These factors include stenting of small vessels, multiple lesions, ostial or bifurcation lesions, suboptimal stent result, heart failure, advanced age, obesity, renal failure, and diabetes. In the presence of these risk factors, the recommended duration is usually prolonged beyond 1 year. Coronary thrombosis after stent implantation has become a rare (0.6%–1.3%) but potentially catastrophic event resulting in an MI and even death (in 25%–45% of cases).[33,34] ASA therapy is usually continued for life.

WITHDRAWAL

Surgeons are faced with decisions as whether to withdraw antiplatelet therapy, on a daily basis. However, stopping or withholding this treatment is associated with increased adverse cardiac, vascular, and ischemic events. In fact, Biondi-Zoccai and colleagues[35] have showed that the cardiac complication rate was 3 times higher after ASA withdrawal and increased even more in patients with coronary stents: ASA cessation is associated with an increased risk of cardiac complications (odds ratio [OR] = 3.1), which peaks at 10 days. This risk is higher after coronary stent placement (OR = 90),[35] especially with drug-eluting stents. Actually, cases of acute thrombosis from drug-eluting stents have been reported with ASA withdrawal beyond 2 years after stent implantation.[36,37] The mean delay between ASA withdrawal and late thrombosis from drug-eluting stents is 7 days.[38] Acute withdrawal of antiplatelet agents produces a deleterious rebound

Table 1 Recommended duration of antiplatelet therapy after a coronary event or intervention	
Coronary Event/ Intervention	**Therapy Type and Duration**
Simple angioplasty without stenting	ASA lifelong
PCI with bare-metal stents	DAPT for 4 wk, then ASA lifelong
MI: medical management	DAPT for 1 y, then ASA lifelong
ACS (unstable)	DAPT for 1 y, then ASA lifelong
PCI with drug-eluting stents	DAPT for 1 y, then ASA lifelong

Abbreviations: DAPT, dual antiplatelet therapy; PCI, percutaneous coronary intervention.

effect: prothrombotic effects overcome the physiologic balance. In fact, excessive thromboxane A2 activity and decreased fibrinolysis have been noted when ASA was stopped. Therefore, the current recommendation is to continue ASA therapy for life. Ideally, this therapy should never be interrupted.

Clopidogrel cessation is the most significant independent predictor of stent thrombosis, with an OR of 14 to 57 during the first 18 months after drug-eluting stent implantation.[39] In fact, premature clopidogrel discontinuation was associated with a hazard ratio of 57.13 (P<.001) and a mortality linked to stent thrombosis of 45%.[34] Ideally, clopidogrel therapy should not be interrupted up to 1 year following the implantation of a drug-eluting stent and 4 weeks following a bare-metal stent because of the increased risk of stent thrombosis.

The perioperative period is usually associated with increased platelet aggregation. Thus, interruption of antiplatelet therapy is riskier in that period. Dual antiplatelet therapy should not be altered during the first 4 weeks after angioplasty and stenting. In fact, stopping this therapy leads to a cardiovascular mortality of up to 71%. Mortality is inversely related to the delay between revascularization and surgery.[40–43] In addition, rebound platelet reactivity after discontinuation of antithrombotic therapy has been shown to lead to increased thrombotic risk in stented patients undergoing surgery.

If antiplatelet therapy is stopped, the recommendation is to discontinue these medications for 5 to 7 days (7 days for prasugrel) before an involved surgical procedure. If patients are at high risk, the recommendation is for a bridging therapy. The ideal bridging agent should be effective in achieving platelet inhibition similar to that of the oral antiplatelets, with a rapid onset of action and a short duration of action. Evidence on the efficacy and safety of short-acting antithrombotic drugs, such as unfractionated heparin, low-molecular-weight heparin (LMWH), or short-acting glycoprotein IIb/IIIa inhibitors (eg, tirofiban, eptifibatide), in the perioperative setting is sparse. However, the authors think that if bridging is necessary, antiplatelet agents should be preferred over anticoagulants, because platelet accumulation at sites of vascular injury is the primary event in arterial thrombosis. If an IV glycoprotein IIb/IIIa inhibitor is used, the infusion should be started 3 days before the surgical procedure and is usually stopped 4 hours before surgery (8 hours in the case of creatinine clearance <30 mL/min). The oral antiplatelet therapy should be resumed within 24 to 48 hours after surgery. As discussed earlier, glycoprotein IIb/IIIa inhibitors have potent antiplatelet effects and are associated with an increased risk of bleeding during their infusion.

HEMORRHAGIC VERSUS THROMBOTIC RISKS

For patients on antiplatelet therapy, surgeons must assess the hemorrhagic risk of the surgical procedure to the thrombotic risk if such therapy is interrupted. Although there is a lack of randomized clinical trials comparing the effects of withdrawing versus continuing antiplatelet agents in the perioperative period, Burger and colleagues[44] have shown that the average relative increase in bleeding during noncardiac surgery is 20% with ASA or clopidogrel alone. However, some operations have an increased risk of postoperative bleeding. These operations include tonsillectomy, transurethral prostatectomy, and intracranial surgery. In fact, after tonsillectomy, the reoperation rate for postoperative hemorrhage was increased 7.2 times in the ASA group compared with the acetaminophen one. Life-threatening hemorrhage has only been reported with intracranial neurosurgical procedures and was actually the major contributing factor of fatal outcomes.[45–48]

Most studies have shown that ASA therapy does not result in increased complication rates. In fact, a meta-analysis comparing surgical bleeding of patients operated on with or without ASA reported no change in the mortality and complication rates. The relative risk of hemorrhage increased up to 50% with dual antiplatelet therapy. Although hemostasis is longer and more difficult to achieve, the surgical mortality and long-term morbidity are not increased.[49–51] In fact, dual antiplatelet therapy does not increase the likelihood of other surgical complications, except for surgeries involving a closed space (eg, intracranial surgery, surgery of the spinal canal, and surgery of the posterior ocular chamber).

Perioperative MI and mortality are actually increased if antiplatelet therapy is withdrawn. In fact, in patients with stents who are on continuous dual antiplatelet therapy, the combined rate of perioperative MI and mortality is the same as in stable CAD. However, withdrawing antiplatelet therapy is associated with a 5- to 10-fold increase in the risk of MI (20%–40%) and mortality (20%–85%), depending on the delay between revascularization and surgery. Therefore, the risk of stent thrombosis appears higher than the risk of surgical hemorrhage, and preoperative cessation of antiplatelet therapy should be avoided when possible. The decision must be made on a case-by-case basis and consultation must be performed with the internist, cardiologist, anesthesiologist, vascular surgeon, and maxillofacial surgeon, after weighing all of the risk factors. Some of the risk factors include the following[52]:

- Coronary status: high risk versus low risk
- Patient's medical status: age, comorbidities
- Extent of PVD
- Type and extent of surgery
- Anticipated blood loss
- Time after stent implantation

WHAT THE ORAL AND MAXILLOFACIAL SURGEON NEEDS TO KNOW

Oral and maxillofacial surgeons are faced with patients on antiplatelet therapy on a daily basis. In fact, most of the current literature supports the continuation of the antiplatelet treatment, especially for minor oral surgical procedures. Cañigral and colleagues[53] conducted a study involving simple and surgical extractions in patients on antiplatelet therapy. The therapy included ASA, clopidogrel, dual antiplatelet therapy (ASA and clopidogrel), nonsteroidal anti-inflammatory drugs, or LMWH. Most surgical bleeding was stopped with local measures. In fact, in 92% of cases, bleeding was stopped within 10 minutes with pressure alone, and 8% of cases were easily managed by local hemostatic measures. Brennan and colleagues[54] reviewed the literature regarding the management of patients on ASA requiring oral surgical procedures. They also recommended continuation of ASA during dental extractions. Gaspar and colleagues[55] concluded that outpatient oral and maxillofacial surgical procedures can be safely performed in patients on ASA therapy, because hemostasis posed no concerns. Their recommendation was to continue ASA therapy without interruption before ambulatory oral surgical procedures. The Oral Medicine and Oral Surgery Francophone Society conducted a literature review and concluded that interruption of antiplatelet therapy before dental procedures is unnecessary and that the risk of bleeding is very low.[56] A recent consensus opinion from the American Heart Association, Society for Cardiovascular Angiography and Interventions, American College of Cardiology, American College of Surgeons, and American Dental Association recommends either continuing dual antiplatelet therapy for minor elective oral surgical procedures in patients who have coronary artery stents or, if possible, delaying treatment until the prescribed regimen is completed.[30]

As discussed earlier, bleeding with ASA does not present a major problem. Matocha[57] reports that the risk of bleeding after dental extractions

is rare in patients on low-dose ASA therapy. In fact, the incidence of bleeding complication after extraction does not exceed 0.2% to 2.3%. Napeñas and colleagues[58,59] evaluated the risk of bleeding in patients on single or dual antiplatelet therapy undergoing invasive oral surgical procedures. The study concluded that the risk of stopping or disrupting antiplatelet therapy and predisposing the patient to thromboembolic events far outweighs the risk of bleeding from a dental procedure. Ardekian and colleagues[60] assessed the risk of bleeding after tooth extraction with the use of ASA (100 mg/d). They found that bleeding was a complication in both patients who stopped ASA and patients who continued ASA therapy. In fact, the bleeding incidence between the 2 groups was comparable, and the hemostasis was easily achieved with local hemostatic measures. Although dual antiplatelet treatment may increase the bleeding risk, the risk of fatal outcomes is generally higher if treatment is stopped and/or altered.[61] Allard and colleagues[62] recommended continuing ASA or clopidogrel in cases involving simple oral surgical procedures. Hemelik and colleagues[63] reviewed the risk of bleeding of 65 patients treated with 100 mg/d of ASA therapy who had extractions. They found that the frequency of postoperative bleeding was minimal and similar in both groups. In addition, all bleeding episodes were easily controlled. They concluded that there is no need to stop 100 mg/d ASA before dental extractions. Krishnan and colleagues[64] concluded that patients on ASA therapy can safely undergo extractions without increased risk of excessive or prolonged postoperative bleeding.

Based on the above studies, the current recommendations are in favor of not stopping antiplatelet treatment with ASA before tooth extraction. Stopping ASA therapy predisposes patients to an increased risk of thromboembolism at the expense of minor intraoperative and/or postoperative bleeding, which can be easily controlled with local measures.

Clinical studies have discussed antiplatelet therapy and its bleeding risk. Napeñas and colleagues[65] reviewed the literature for bleeding complications after dental procedures in patients on antiplatelet therapy. They found 15 studies involving 2428 patients who were on ASA, clopidogrel, cilostazol, dipyridamole, ticlopidine, and/or triflusal. The study concluded that although there appeared to be an increased occurrence of minor immediate postoperative bleeding, there were no clinically significant increases in the frequency and degree of intraoperative as well as postoperative bleeding complications. The

Table 2
Risk of procedures with regards to antiplatelet therapy

Procedures	Examples	Antiplatelet Therapy	Dual Antiplatelet Therapy
Low risk	• Single extraction • Soft tissue biopsy/excision of soft tissue lesion ≤1 cm in diameter	• No change • Local hemostatic measures	• No change • Local hemostatic measures
Medium risk	• Multiple extractions: ≤5 teeth • Soft tissue biopsy/excision of soft tissue lesion 1–3 cm in diameter • Placement of 1–3 dental implants	• No change • Local hemostatic measures	• Consider withdrawal of one of the drugs before procedure (depending on patient's risk factors) • Restart after hemostasis is achieved
High risk	• Multiple extractions: >5 teeth • Surgical extractions of impacted teeth (eg, impacted wisdom teeth) • Soft tissue biopsy/excision of soft tissue lesion >3 cm • Biopsy/excision of a hard tissue lesion • Removal of maxillary and/or mandibular tori • Placement of multiple dental implants: >3 implants	• No change • Local hemostatic measures	• Withhold one of the drugs before procedure • Restart after hemostasis is achieved

procedures evaluated included simple and surgical extractions, deep scaling, endodontic procedures, biopsies, periodontal surgery, and surgical placement of dental implants. The rationale for maintenance of antiplatelet therapy during oral and maxillofacial surgical procedures is also supported by the widely accepted opinion that the cardioprotective benefit of antiplatelet therapy far outweighs the potential risk of bleeding.[66] **Table 2** summarizes the authors' recommendations.

Antiplatelet therapy is safe for most maxillofacial trauma patients, except patients who present with orbital floor fractures. In fact, severe bleeding and increased risk of retrobulbar hematomas have occurred in patients with orbital fractures on antiplatelet or anticoagulant therapy.[67] The risk of hematoma formation is actually increased in orbital or skull base surgery in patients on antiplatelet therapy.

SUMMARY

Most patients with CAD and PVD are on long-term antiplatelet therapy and dual therapy. Knowledge and understanding of the mechanism of action of these different agents will allow us to treat our patients safely and minimize the risk of adverse events. Achieving the fine balance between ischemic and bleeding risk remains a challenge in patients undergoing surgery who are treated with

antiplatelet therapy. Finally, for most of our outpatient surgical procedures, maintenance and continuation of this therapy are recommended. Consultation with the patient's cardiologist, physician, and/or vascular surgeon is always recommended before interrupting this treatment modality.

REFERENCES

1. Zorprin, Bayer Buffered Aspirin (aspirin) dosing, indications, interactions, adverse effects, and more. Medscape Reference. Accessed February 29, 2016. Available at: http://reference.medscape.com/drug/zorprin-bayer-buffered-aspirin-343279.
2. Brayfield A, editor. Aspirin. Martindale: the complete drug reference. Pharmaceutical Press; 2014. Accessed March 2, 2016 Available at: https://www.medicinescomplete.com/mc/martindale/current/login.htm?uri=https%3A%2F%2Fwww.medicinescomplete.com%2Fmc%2Fmartindale%2Fcurrent%2F2601-s.htm.
3. Manzano A, Pérez-Segura P. Colorectal cancer chemoprevention: is this the future of colorectal cancer prevention? ScientificWorldJournal 2012;2012:327341.
4. Chan AT, Arber N, Burn J, et al. Aspirin in the chemoprevention of colorectal neoplasia: an overview. Cancer Prev Res (Phila) 2012;5(2):164–78.
5. Thun MJ, Jacobs EJ, Patrono C. The role of aspirin in cancer prevention. Nat Rev Clin Oncol 2012;9(5):259–67.

6. Verdoodt F, Friis S, Dehlendorff C, et al. Non-steroidal anti-inflammatory drug use and risk of endometrial cancer: a systematic review and meta-analysis of observational studies. Gynecol Oncol 2016; 140(2):352–8.

7. Randomised trial of intravenous streptokinase, oral aspirin, both, or neither among 17,187 cases of suspected acute myocardial infarction: ISIS-2. ISIS-2 (Second International Study of Infarct Survival) Collaborative Group. Lancet 1988;2:349–60.

8. Collaborative overview of randomized trials of antiplatelet treatment, I: prevention of vascular death, MI and stroke by prolonged antiplatelet therapy in different categories of patients. Antiplatelet Trialists Collaboration. Br Med J 1994;308:235–46.

9. O'Gara PT, Kushner FG, Ascheim DD, Casey DE, Chung MK, de Lemos JA, et al. 2013 ACCF/AHA guideline for the management of ST-elevation myocardial infarction: a report of the American College of Cardiology Foundation/American Heart Association Task Force on Practice Guidelines. J Am Coll Cardiol 2013;61(4):e78–140.

10. Jneid H, Anderson JL, Wright RS, et al. 2012 ACCF/AHA focused update of the guideline for the management of patients with unstable angina/non-ST-elevation myocardial infarction (updating the 2007 guideline and replacing the 2011 focused update): a report of the American College of Cardiology Foundation/American Heart Association Task Force on practice guidelines. Circulation 2012;126(7): 875–910.

11. Fihn SD, Gardin JM, Abrams J, et al. 2012 ACCF/AHA/ACP/AATS/PCNA/SCAI/STS guideline for the diagnosis and management of patients with stable ischemic heart disease: executive summary: a report of the American College of Cardiology Foundation/American Heart Association task force on practice guidelines, and the American College of Physicians, American Association for Thoracic Surgery, Preventive Cardiovascular Nurses Association, Society for Cardiovascular Angiography and Interventions, and Society of Thoracic Surgeons. Circulation 2012;126(25):3097–137.

12. Rossi S, editor. Australian medicines handbook 2006. Adelaide (South Australia): Australian Medicines Handbook; 2006.

13. Wedemeyer RS, Blume H. Pharmacokinetic drug interaction profiles of proton pump inhibitors: an update. Drug Saf 2014;37(4):201–11.

14. Brown DG, Wilkerson EC, Love WE. A review of traditional and novel oral anticoagulant and antiplatelet therapy for dermatologists and dermatologic surgeons. J Am Acad Dermatol 2015;72(3):524–34.

15. Pereillo JM, Maftouh M, Andrieu A, et al. Structure and stereochemistry of the active metabolite of clopidogrel (PDF). Drug Metab Dispos 2002;30(11): 1288–95.

16. Mega JL, Close SL, Wiviott SD, et al. Cytochrome p-450 polymorphisms and response to clopidogrel. N Engl J Med 2009;360(4):354–62.

17. Simon T, Verstuyft C, Mary-Krause M, et al. Genetic determinants of response to clopidogrel and cardiovascular events. N Engl J Med 2009;360(4):363–75.

18. Collet JP, Hulot JS, Pena A, et al. Cytochrome P450 2C19 polymorphism in young patients treated with clopidogrel after myocardial infarction: a cohort study. Lancet 2009;373(9660):309–17.

19. Baker WL, White CM. Role of prasugrel, a novel P2Y(12) receptor antagonist, in the management of acute coronary syndromes. Am J Cardiovasc Drugs 2009;9(4):213–29.

20. Wallentin L, Becker RC, Budaj A, PLATO Investigators. Ticagrelor versus clopidogrel in patients with acute coronary syndromes. N Engl J Med 2009; 361:1045–57.

21. Bonaca MP, Bhatt DL, Cohen M. PEGASUS-TIMI 54 Steering Committee and Investigators. Long-term use of ticagrelor in patients with prior myocardial infarction. N Engl J Med 2015;372:1791–800.

22. Hiatt WR. Medical treatment of peripheral arterial disease and claudication. N Engl J Med 2001;344: 1608–21.

23. Aniguchi K, Ohtani H, Ikemoto T, et al. Possible case of potentiation of the antiplatelet effect of cilostazol by grapefruit juice. J Clin Pharm Ther 2007;32(5): 457–9.

24. Dixon BS, Beck GJ, Vazquez MA, et al. Effect of dipyridamole plus aspirin on hemodialysis graft patency. N Engl J Med 2009;360(21):2191–201.

25. Use of a monoclonal antibody directed against the platelet glycoprotein IIb/IIIa receptor in high-risk coronary angioplasty. The EPIC Investigation. N Engl J Med 1994;330(14):956–61.

26. Inhibition of platelet glycoprotein IIb/IIIa with eptifibatide in patients with acute coronary syndromes. The PURSUIT Trial Investigators. Platelet glycoprotein IIb/IIIa in unstable angina: receptor suppression using integrilin therapy. N Engl J Med 1998;339: 436–43.

27. Inhibition of the platelet glycoprotein IIb/IIIa receptor with tirofiban in unstable angina and non-Q-wave myocardial infarction. Platelet Receptor Inhibition in Ischemic Syndrome Management in Patients Limited by Unstable Signs and Symptoms (PRISM-PLUS) Study Investigators. N Engl J Med 1998; 338:1488–97.

28. Joner M, Finn AV, Farb A, et al. Pathology of drug-eluting stents in humans: delayed healing and late thrombotic risk. J Am Coll Cardiol 2006;48(1):193–202.

29. Eberli D, Chassot PG, Sulser T, et al. Urological surgery and antiplatelet drugs after cardiac and cerebrovascular accidents. J Urol 2010;183(6): 2128–36.

30. Grines CL, Bonow RO, Casey DE Jr, et al. Prevention of premature discontinuation of dual antiplatelet therapy in patients with coronary artery stents: a science advisory from the American Heart Association, American College of Cardiology, Society for Cardiovascular Angiography and Interventions, American College of Surgeons, and American Dental Association, with representation from the American College of Physicians. Circulation 2007;115(6):813–8.

31. American Society of Anesthesiologists Committee on Standards and Practice Parameters. Practice alert for the perioperative management of patients with coronary artery stents: a report by the American Society of Anesthesiologists Committee on Standards and Practice Parameters. Anesthesiology 2009;110(1):22–3.

32. Douketis JD, Berger PB, Dunn AS, et al. The perioperative management of antithrombotic therapy: American College of Chest Physicians Evidence-Based Clinical Practice Guidelines (8th edition). Chest 2008;133(6 suppl):299S–339S.

33. Daemen J, Wenaweser P, Tsuchida K, et al. Early and late coronary stent thrombosis of sirolimus-eluting and paclitaxel-eluting stents in routine clinical practice: data from a large two-institutional cohort study. Lancet 2007;369(9562):667–78.

34. Iakovou I, Schmidt T, Bonizzoni E, et al. Incidence, predictors, and outcome of thrombosis after successful implantation of drug-eluting stents. JAMA 2005;293(17):2126–30.

35. Biondi-Zoccai GG, Lotrionte M, Agostoni P, et al. A systematic review and meta-analysis on the hazards of discontinuing or not adhering to aspirin among 50,279 patients at risk for coronary artery disease. Eur Heart J 2006;27(22):2667–74.

36. Artang R, Dieter RS. Analysis of 36 reported cases of late thrombosis in drug-eluting stents placed in coronary arteries. Am J Cardiol 2007; 99(8):1039–43.

37. de Souza DG, Baum VC, Ballert NM. Late thrombosis of a drug-eluting stent presenting in the perioperative period. Anesthesiology 2007;106(5): 1057–9.

38. Eisenberg MJ, Richard PR, Libersan D, et al. Safety of short-term discontinuation of antiplatelet therapy in patients with drug-eluting stents. Circulation 2009;119(12):1634–42.

39. Airoldi F, Colombo A, Morici N, et al. Incidence and predictors of drug-eluting stent thrombosis during and after discontinuation of thienopyridine treatment. Circulation 2007;116(7):745–54.

40. Sharma AK, Ajani AE, Hamwi SM, et al. Major noncardiac surgery following coronary stenting: when is it safe to operate? Catheter Cardiovasc Interv 2004;63(2):141–5.

41. Nuttall GA, Brown MJ, Stombaugh JW, et al. Time and cardiac risk of surgery after bare-metal stent percutaneous coronary intervention. Anesthesiology 2008;109(4):588–95.

42. Rabbitts JA, Nuttall GA, Brown MJ, et al. Cardiac risk of noncardiac surgery after percutaneous coronary intervention with drug-eluting stents. Anesthesiology 2008;109(4):596–604.

43. Schouten O, van Domburg RT, Bax JJ, et al. Noncardiac surgery after coronary stenting: early surgery and interruption of antiplatelet therapy are associated with an increase in major adverse cardiac events. J Am Coll Cardiol 2007;49(1): 122–4.

44. Burger W, Chemnitius JM, Kneissl GD, et al. Low-dose aspirin for secondary cardiovascular prevention - cardiovascular risks after its perioperative withdrawal versus bleeding risks with its continuation - review and meta-analysis. J Intern Med 2005; 257(5):399–414.

45. Stage J, Jensen JH, Bonding P. Post-tonsillectomy haemorrhage and analgesics. A comparative study of acetylsalicylic acid and paracetamol. Clin Otolaryngol Allied Sci 1988;13(3):201–4.

46. Nielsen JD, Holm-Nielsen A, Jespersen J, et al. The effect of low-dose acetylsalicylic acid on bleeding after transurethral prostatectomy—a prospective, randomized, double-blind, placebo-controlled study. Scand J Urol Nephrol 2000;34(3):194–8.

47. Halliwell OT, Yadegafar G, Lane C, et al. Transrectal ultrasound-guided biopsy of the prostate: aspirin increases the incidence of minor bleeding complications. Clin Radiol 2008;63(5):557–61.

48. Palmer JD, Sparrow OC, Iannotti F. Postoperative hematoma: a 5-year survey identification of avoidable risk factors. Neurosurgery 1994;35:1061–4.

49. Chapman TW, Bowley DM, Lambert AW, et al. Haemorrhage associated with combined clopidogrel and aspirin therapy. Eur J Vasc Endovasc Surg 2001;22(5):478–9.

50. Moore M, Power M. Perioperative hemorrhage and combined clopidogrel and aspirin therapy. Anesthesiology 2004;101(3):792–4.

51. Ernst A, Eberhardt R, Wahidi M, et al. Effect of routine clopidogrel use on bleeding complications after transbronchial biopsy in humans. Chest 2006; 129(3):734–7.

52. Chassot PG, Delabays A, Spahn DR. Perioperative antiplatelet therapy: the case for continuing therapy in patients at risk of myocardial infarction. Br J Anaesth 2007;99(3):316–28.

53. Cañigral A, Silvestre F-J, Cañigral G, et al. Evaluation of bleeding risk and measurement methods in dental patients. Med Oral Patol Oral Cir Bucal 2010;15(6):e863–8.

54. Brennan MT, Wynn RL, Miller CS. Aspirin and bleeding in dentistry: an update and recommendations. Oral Surg Oral Med Oral Pathol Oral Radiol Endod 2007;104(3):316–23.

55. Gaspar R, Ardekian L, Brenner B, et al. Ambulatory oral procedures on low-dose aspirin. Harefuah 1999; 136(2):108–10.

56. Oral Medicine and Oral Surgery Francophone Society, Management of patients under anti-platelet agents' treatment in odotostomatology. Available at: http://www.mbcb-journal.org/images/stories/recommendations/recommandations_antiplaquetalres_en.pdf. Accessed March 2, 2016.

57. Matocha DL. Postsurgical complications. Emerg Med Clin North Am 2000;18(3):549–64.

58. Murphy J, Twohig E, McWilliams SR. Dentists' approach to patients on anti-platelet agents and warfarin: a survey of practice. J Ir Dent Assoc 2010;56(1):28–31.

59. Napeñas J, Hong CHL, Brennan MT, et al. The frequency of bleeding complications after invasive dental treatment in patients receiving single and dual antiplatelet therapy. J Am Dent Assoc 2009; 140(6):690–5.

60. Ardekian L, Gaspar R, Peled M, et al. Does low-dose aspirin therapy complicate oral surgical procedures? J Am Dent Assoc 2000;131(3): 331–5.

61. Nielsen JD, Lætgaard CA, Schou S, et al. Minor dentoalveolar surgery in patients undergoing antithrombotic therapy. Ugeskr Laeger 2009; 171(17):1407–9.

62. Allard RH, Baart JA, Huijgens PC, et al. Antithrombotic therapy and dental surgery with bleeding. Ned Tijdschr Tandheelkd 2004;111(12):482–5.

63. Hemelik M, Wahl G, Kessler B. Tooth extraction under medication with acetylsalicylic acid. Mund Kiefer Gesichtschir 2006;10(1):3–6.

64. Krishnan B, Shenoy NA, Alexander M. Exodontia and antiplatelet therapy. J Oral Maxillofac Surg 2008;66(10):2063–6.

65. Napennas JJ, Oost FC, DeGroot A, et al. Review of postoperative bleeding risk in dental patients on antiplatelet therapy. Oral Surg Oral Med Oral Pathol Oral Radiol 2013;115:491–9.

66. Antithrombotic Trialists' Collaboration. Collaborative meta-analysis of randomised trials of antiplatelet therapy for prevention of death, myocardial infarction, and stroke in high risk patients. BMJ 2002; 324:71–86.

67. Maurer P, Conrad-Hengerer I, Hollstein S, et al. Orbital haemorrhage associated with orbital fractures in geriatric patients on antiplatelet or anticoagulant therapy. Int J Oral Maxillofac Surg 2013;42(12): 1510–4.

Heparin and Lovenox
What the Oral and Maxillofacial Surgeon Needs to Know

LisaMarie Di Pasquale, DDS, MD[a],
Elie M. Ferneini, DMD, MD, MHS, MBA[b,c,*]

KEYWORDS

- Heparin • Lovenox • Fondaparinux • Anticoagulation • Protamine sulfate

KEY POINTS

- Many of our surgical patients are on heparin products during surgery.
- There is no standardized approach to treating anticoagulated patients during oral and maxillofacial surgical procedures.
- When a patient is on heparin therapy, heparin may be stopped 4 to 6 hours before the surgical procedure and resumed once hemostasis is achieved (usually within 24 hours).
- If low-molecular-weight heparin is given, the treatment is generally stopped at least 12 hours before surgery and then resumed once hemostasis is achieved.

INTRODUCTION

Heparin is a naturally occurring glycosaminoglycan anticoagulant found in the secretory granules of mast cells. It is composed of alternating D-glucuronic acid and N-acetyl-D-glucosamine residues.[1] Following synthesis inside the mast cell, a glucuronidase enzyme slowly degrades the glycosaminoglycan chains to various-sized heparin fragments.[2,3] *Unfractionated heparin* is a term for the heterogeneous heparin molecules that have not been separated according to length, which can vary between 5 and 30 kD. By itself, heparin has no intrinsic anticoagulant effect. Antithrombin is a serine protease inhibitor that inhibits several coagulation factors in the intrinsic and common pathway.[2] Antithrombin binds to a specific 5-saccharide sequence on heparin. When antithrombin binds heparin, a conformational change is induced within the antithrombin enzyme. This activated antithrombin then binds coagulation factor Xa with increased affinity and accelerates its inactivation.[2–4] Thrombin (factor II) inhibition occurs when antithrombin and thrombin bind concurrently to adjacent sites on a heparin molecule. Only heparin molecules at least 18-saccharide units long are able to bind both thrombin and antithrombin simultaneously.[3] Heparin then acts as a catalyst to facilitate thrombin binding to antithrombin, forming a ternary complex that causes thrombin inhibition. Interestingly, because of their variety in fragment size, not all heparin molecules have anticoagulant activity. Some molecules may be missing the necessary 5-saccharide sequence required to bind antithrombin, whereas the chains less than 18-saccharide units are not able to span antithrombin and thrombin together to cause thrombin inhibition.[3,4]

[a] Division of Oral and Maxillofacial Surgery, Department of Craniofacial Sciences, University of Connecticut, 263 Farmington Avenue, Farmington, CT 06030, USA; [b] Private Practice, Greater Waterbury OMS, 435 Highland Avenue, Suite 100, Cheshire, CT 06410, USA; [c] Beau Visage Med Spa, 435 Highland Avenue, Suite 100, Cheshire, CT 06410, USA
* Corresponding author.
E-mail address: eferneini@yahoo.com

Oral Maxillofacial Surg Clin N Am 28 (2016) 507–513
http://dx.doi.org/10.1016/j.coms.2016.06.008

Low-molecular-weight heparins (LMWHs), trade name Lovenox, are derivatives of heparin used for anticoagulation. LMWHs are produced by chemically decreasing the number of the polysaccharide units on heparin, resulting in molecules that average 4 to 5 kD in weight. LMWHs that possess the necessary 5-saccharide chain retain the ability to bind antithrombin and inactivate factor Xa, as described for heparin.[3] LMWHs have inherently less antithrombin activity, however, because they are not of sufficient length to form the ternary complex bridging thrombin to antithrombin for inactivation.[3,5] **Fig. 1** compares the mechanism of action of heparin with LMWH and fondaparinux.

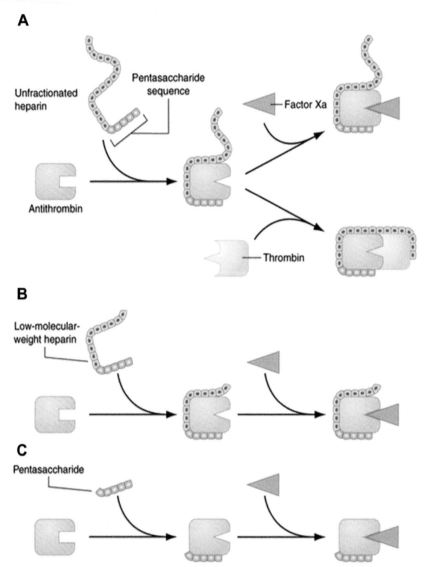

Fig. 1. Mechanism of action of heparin, LMWH, and fondaparinux, a synthetic pentasaccharide. (*A*) Heparin binds to antithrombin via its pentasaccharide sequence. This binding induces a conformational change in the reactive center loop of antithrombin that accelerates its interaction with factor Xa. To potentiate thrombin inhibition, heparin must simultaneously bind to antithrombin and thrombin. Only heparin chains composed of at least 18 saccharide units, which correspond to a molecular weight of 5400 Da, are of sufficient length to perform this bridging function. With a mean molecular weight of 15,000 Da, all of the heparin chains are long enough to do this. (*B*) LMWH has greater capacity to potentiate factor Xa inhibition by antithrombin than thrombin because, with a mean molecular weight of 4500 to 5000 Da, at least half of the LMWH chains are too short to bridge antithrombin to thrombin. (*C*) The pentasaccharide only accelerates factor Xa inhibition by antithrombin because the pentasaccharide is too short to bridge antithrombin to thrombin. *From* Kasper D, Fauci A, Hauser S, et al, editors. Harrison's principles of internal medicine. 19th edition. New York: McGraw-Hill; 2015; with permission.

USES

There are many medical and surgical uses for heparin products. Heparin has a rapid onset time, so it is used to prevent thrombus formation and therapeutically to stop extension of an existing thrombus. Thus, heparin is the first-line agent for treating postoperative deep venous thrombosis and pulmonary embolism.[2,5] Heparin products are also widely used in cardiac patients, often in the regimen for the management of unstable angina or acute myocardial infarction. Additionally, patients with cardiac dysrhythmias, such as atrial fibrillation, will typically be started on heparin for the purposes of preventing thromboembolic disease.[3,4] Other medical uses of heparin include treatment of a variety of prothrombotic conditions, including disseminated intravascular coagulation (DIC); deficiencies of protein C, protein S, and antithrombin; elevated levels of homocysteine; certain cancers; antiphospholipid antibody syndrome; and factor V Leiden gene mutations.[2] In the operating room, heparin anticoagulation is used during cardiopulmonary bypass, with the effect of the drug easily reversible with protamine sulfate after the procedure.[5]

PHARMACOLOGY/PHARMACOKINETICS

The pharmacologic properties of heparin vary among individual patients and depend on the route of administration. Heparin is not absorbed after oral ingestion, so it must be given parenterally.[2] Heparin is administered by continuous intravenous infusion, intermittent infusion, or subcutaneous injection.[5] Heparin has an immediate onset of action following parenteral administration. However, there is a wide variability in the bioavailability of heparin, as it binds to plasma proteins and other cells.[3] This causes a dose-dependent half-life that can vary from 1 to 2 hours. The short chains of the LMWHs exhibit less cellular interactions than unfractionated heparin and, consequently, result in a more predictable dose response.[4] LMWH also has a longer half-life, around 4 hours, and can be administered once or twice daily by a subcutaneous route.[5] Heparin is primarily metabolized by the liver and then cleared by the kidneys, although interaction and degradation by macrophages in the reticuloendothelial system does occur.[3]

DOSING

Heparin is usually administered subcutaneously or by intravenous infusion. As it is not absorbed orally, it must be given parenterally. To achieve a full effect rapidly, full-dose therapeutic heparin is typically administered by continuous intravenous infusion. Following an initial bolus of 5000 U or 80 U/kg, therapeutic heparin is then infused at a rate of 12 to 18 U/kg/h.[5] Fixed-dose or weight-based heparin nomograms exist in attempts to standardize therapeutic heparin dosing. Weight-based heparin dosages tend to be more rapid and more effective in achieving therapeutic anticoagulation than fixed-dose boluses.[4] With continuous intravenous infusions, due to the erratic bioavailability of heparin, frequent anticoagulation monitoring is necessary; the dose can be adjusted to obtain a therapeutic level.[2] Heparin can also be administered therapeutically via a subcutaneous route on a twice-daily basis. A typical daily dose of 35,000 U is divided into twice-daily administrations to achieve therapeutic values similar to that of intravenous heparin.[5]

LMWHs have distinct biological advantages for treatment purposes. The more predictable dose response permits therapeutic subcutaneous dosing 1 to 2 times daily in fixed or weight-adjusted doses without the need for coagulation monitoring.[4] Therapeutic LMWH is administered by a dose of 1.5 to 2.0 mg/kg if the drug is administered once daily. Otherwise, a LMWH dosage of 1 mg/kg every 12 hours is sufficient for treatment.[5]

For prophylaxis, heparin is usually given in fixed doses of 5000 U subcutaneously 2 or 3 times daily. With these low doses, coagulation monitoring is thought to be unnecessary.[3] The prophylactic doses of LMWH can vary; a once-daily subcutaneous dose of 40 mg can be given, or LMWH can be administered twice daily with doses of 25 to 30 mg.[5] Often, for patients who will require long-term therapy, heparin or LMWH is started initially to promote therapeutic anticoagulation. Treatment with a vitamin K antagonist is then overlapped for 4 to 5 days, and heparin is discontinued once therapeutic anticoagulation is achieved.[4]

MONITORING

Heparin therapy can be monitored using the activated partial thromboplastin time (aPTT) or anti–factor Xa level. The usual therapeutic range for aPTT during heparin therapy is between 1.5 and 2.5 times the normal range.[2] Although the anticoagulant effect is immediate, laboratory monitoring is absolutely essential when the drug is given in therapeutic doses. In contrast, for prophylactic uses, heparin is usually given in fixed low doses subcutaneously and monitoring is unnecessary.[3]

Alternatively, monitoring can be performed using anti–factor Xa levels, which is useful if the aPTT is unreliable. With this test, therapeutic heparin levels range from 0.3 to 0.7 U/mL when measured 3 to 4 hours after drug administration.[2] In general, because of less variability in the chain size, LMWHs produce a more predictable dose response than unfractionated heparin. Therefore, monitoring is not routinely done. Nonetheless, the therapeutic anti–factor Xa levels generally range from 0.5 to 1.2 U/mL. When LMWH is given strictly for prophylactic doses, anti–factor Xa levels of 0.2 to 0.5 U/mL are preferred.[4]

SIDE EFFECTS

The most frequent complication of heparin administration is bleeding, which is related to the dose and intensity of treatment as well as to patient factors. Concomitant administration of drugs that affect hemostasis, such as antiplatelet or fibrinolytic agents, increases the risk of bleeding, as does recent surgery or trauma. Major bleeding is defined as bleeding that results in a decrease of hemoglobin at least 2 g/dL or requires transfusion of at least 2 U of packed red cells.[1] The rate of major bleeding is generally low, 1% to 2%, when heparin is used for initial treatment. Certain patient factors contribute to bleeding as well, including the concurrent use of particular medications as well as medical conditions with a propensity for bleeding, such as thrombocytopenia and liver disease.[1–4]

Heparin and LMWH may cause thrombocytopenia. Heparin-induced thrombocytopenia (HIT) is caused by circulating immunoglobulin G antibodies against the complexes of heparin with platelet factor 4 and, to a lesser extent, to individual platelets.[4] The defining clinical sign is a decrease in platelet count, generally a 50% decrease from baseline or development of platelet count less than 150,000/μL occurring around day 5 in the course of treatment with heparin.[3] Diagnosis of HIT is confirmed by laboratory tests that identify antiplatelet factor 4 antibodies in patient serum or by serotonin release assays, in which platelets containing labeled serotonin lyse and release serotonin when exposed to heparin and patient serum that is positive for HIT antibody.[4] Despite thrombocytopenia, HIT is usually associated with clot formation and thromboembolic complications.[2] The risk of HIT is about notably lower with LMWH; however, it can occur regardless of the route or type of heparin administration. Because of potential cross reactivity, all heparin products should be discontinued immediately when the diagnosis of HIT is made. Anticoagulation with an alternative nonheparin anticoagulant should be initiated, such as a direct thrombin inhibitor. Further anticoagulation with an oral vitamin K antagonist can be safely resumed once the platelet count has increased to more than 150,000/μL.[3]

Osteoporosis may occur as a result of long-term treatment with heparin products. It is associated with therapeutic range treatment that has been administered for greater than 3 months. Affecting both the function of osteoblasts and osteoclasts, heparin-associated bone loss can cause symptomatic bone and back pain; rarely, vertebral fractures occur in these individuals. Heparin may also be associated with hypoaldosteronism, elevated transaminase levels, and, infrequently, allergic reactions.[1–4]

CONTRAINDICATIONS

The absolute contraindication to anticoagulant treatment is severe, active bleeding. In addition, intracranial hemorrhage, spinal cord surgery, spinal procedures, and severe hypertension would also contraindicate use of anticoagulants.[1] Other relative contraindications may include recent major surgery, recent hemorrhagic cerebrovascular event, severe renal failure, and thrombocytopenia less than 50,000/μL.[1]

LMWHs rely almost exclusively on renal clearance. High levels of LMWH can accumulate in patients with renal insufficiency and cause further bleeding. In this situation, LMWH therapy should be monitored with anti–factor Xa levels.[1] Additionally, the oral and maxillofacial surgeon should be aware of patients with inherited antithrombin deficiency, hepatic cirrhosis, and nephrotic syndrome, in which alterations in the synthesis of coagulation factors and changes in heparin metabolism cause variable pharmacologic effects.[3]

REVERSAL

Heparin has a short half-life, and its anticoagulant effect diminishes within a few hours after discontinuation of the drug.[5] If bleeding during treatment occurs, the infusion is stopped and local measures are usually sufficient to control hemorrhage. However, in the event of major bleeding, the anticoagulant effect can be neutralized with protamine sulfate. Protamine sulfate is a protein that binds the heparin molecule very strongly, and the protamine-heparin complexes are then cleared, neutralizing heparin's anticoagulant effect. The dose required is based on the amount of circulating heparin; usually 1 mg of protamine is required to neutralize 100 units of heparin. Of note, protamine sulfate only binds the longer chains of heparin, thus only has a partial effect on the anti–factor Xa activity of LMWH.[2–5] Protamine can cause widespread histamine release resulting in anaphylactoid reactions. To avoid possible complications of hypotension and pulmonary edema, the drug should be administered slowly and the dosage should not exceed 50 mg intravenously over a 10-minute period.[5] **Table 1** discusses the advantages of LWMH over heparin.

FONDAPARINUX

Fondaparinux is a synthetic five-saccharide chain analogous to the pentasaccharide antithrombin binding sequence found in heparin. Thus, fondaparinux selectively causes inhibition of factor Xa, and has been shown to be as effective and safe as LMWH for the initial treatment of pulmonary embolism and deep vein thrombosis.[2–5] Fondaparinux is administered by weight-based dosing, given subcutaneously once daily at a dose of 5.0 mg for patients weighing less than 50 kg, 7.5 mg for patients weighing between 50 and 100 kg, and 10.0 mg for patients weighing more than 100 kg.[4] Like LMWH, fondaparinux may be monitored using an anti-Xa assay; however, because it does not have significant plasma reactions, it can also be given without coagulation monitoring. The half-life of fondaparinux is the longest of any heparin product, approximately 17 hours; the drug is cleared by the kidneys.[3] Like LMWH, care should be taken in using the drug in patients with renal insufficiency.

MANAGEMENT OF PATIENTS REQUIRING ORAL AND MAXILLOFACIAL SURGERY

For the oral and maxillofacial surgeon, many patients will be on heparin products during surgery. So far, there is no standardized approach to treating anticoagulated patients during oral surgical procedures. It is common for patients who take vitamin K antagonist therapy to bridge their therapy, which is accomplished by discontinuing vitamin K antagonist and switching to either heparin or LMWH. When a patient is on heparin therapy, because of a short half-life, the heparin may be stopped 4 to 6 hours before the surgery and resumed once a stable hemostasis has been established, usually within 24 hours. If LMWH is given, the treatment is generally stopped at least 12 hours before the surgery and then resumed in a similar fashion. Local measures are generally enough to provide adequate hemostasis, although a risk for postoperative hemorrhage, albeit small, does exist.[6–8] Host factors, degree of anticoagulation, and extent of surgery do seem to play a role in the amount of postoperative hemorrhage. In some cases of acute cerebral infarction or acute coronary syndrome, oral surgical procedures may be necessary on patients who are receiving continuous heparin infusions. In these cases, hemostatic control is likely to be a problem. Hemostatic management should be achieved with local measures as best as possible.[8] **Table 2** compares heparin, LMWH, and fondaparinux.

Many procedures in oral and maxillofacial surgery are relatively minor in nature and typically occur in a healthy, active patient base with limited risk factors for the development of thromboembolic disease. However, longer, complex operations do occur and potentially in a less healthy patient base that may be slow to ambulate postoperatively.[7] For thromboembolic prophylaxis during the perioperative period, external compression with graduated elastic compression stockings is generally safe. Chemoprophylaxis with heparin or LMWH is commonly administered when longer, more complicated procedures are performed in patients who may not mobilize

Table 1 Advantages of low-molecular-weight heparin over heparin	
Advantage	**Clinical Significance**
Bioavailability	There is wide variability in the bioavailability of heparin (binds to plasma proteins and other cells). LMWH exhibits less cellular interactions and better bioavailability.
Dosing	Heparin has a dose-dependent half-life. LMWH has a more predictable dose response, so it can be administered 1–2 times daily.
Monitoring	There is erratic bioavailability of heparin; frequent anticoagulation monitoring is necessary (for continuous intravenous infusions). LMWH has a predictable dose response and can dose generally without the need for monitoring.
Side effects	LMWH has less risk of significant bleeding. It is less likely to cause HIT or osteoporosis.

Table 2
Comparison of heparin, low-molecular-weight heparin, and fondaparinux

	Heparin	LMWH	Fondaparinux
Mechanism	Increases AT affinity for Xa, accelerates Xa inhibition Binds simultaneously to AT and thrombin, catalyzes thrombin inhibition	Accelerates Xa inhibition (mechanism analogous to heparin) Less thrombin inhibition (chains too short to bind AT and thrombin simultaneously)	Synthetic analogue of LMWH and selectively inhibits Xa (Like LMWH, only has the AT binding sequence; too short to affect thrombin inhibition)
Half-life	1–2 h	4–6 h	17 h
Monitoring	aPTT for continuous infusion (anti–Xa level if aPTT unreliable)	None (anti–Xa factor can be quantified)	None
Reversal	Protamine sulfate (1 mg neutralizes 100 units of heparin)	Protamine sulfate = only a partial effect on the anti-Xa activity of LMWH (only binds longer chains of heparin)	None
Clearance	Hepatic (also degraded by macrophages in the reticuloendothelial system)	Exclusively renal (adjust dose in renal insufficiency)	Analogous to LMWH
HIT	Causes HIT Do not give to patients within 3 mo of suspected HIT	Can cause HIT (follow guidelines as for heparin)	Does not cause HIT
Last dose before procedure	4–6 h	12–24 h	4–5 d
Pregnancy/ breastfeeding	OK	OK	Insufficient data

Abbreviation: AT, antithrombin.

quickly in the postoperative course.[9] Patient risk factors for thromboembolic events include obesity, hypercoagulability, malignancy, immobility, smoking, and medical history with attention to previous deep vein thrombosis or pulmonary embolism. The decision to use mechanical versus chemoprophylaxis should be assessed in every patient, and balance the risks of thromboembolism versus bleeding in the individual patient.[7,9]

REFERENCES

1. Raskob GE, Hull RD, Pineo GF. Chapter 134. Venous thrombosis. In: Lichtman MA, Kipps TJ, Seligsohn U, et al, editors. Williams hematology. 8th edition. New York: McGraw-Hill; 2010. p. 2185–96. Available at: http://accessmedicine.mhmedical.com.online.uchc.edu/content.aspx?bookid=358&Sectionid=39835958. Accessed August 30, 2015.
2. Francis CW, Crowther M. Chapter 23. Principles of antithrombotic therapy. In: Lichtman MA, Kipps TJ, Seligsohn U, et al, editors. Williams hematology. 8th edition. New York: McGraw-Hill; 2010. p. 353–68. Available at: http://accessmedicine.mhmedical.com.online.uchc.edu/content.aspx?bookid=358&Sectionid=39835840. Accessed August 30, 2015.
3. Weitz JI. Chapter 30. Blood coagulation and anticoagulant, fibrinolytic, and antiplatelet drugs. In: Brunton LL, Chabner BA, Knollmann BC, editors. Goodman & Gilman's the pharmacological basis of therapeutics. 12th edition. New York: McGraw-Hill; 2011. p. 849–76. Available at: http://accessmedicine.mhmedical.com.online.uchc.edu/content.aspx?bookid=374&Sectionid=41266237. Accessed August 30, 2015.
4. Weitz JI. Antiplatelet, anticoagulant, and fibrinolytic drugs. In: Kasper D, Fauci A, Hauser S, et al, editors. Harrison's principles of internal medicine. 19th edition. New York: McGraw-Hill; 2015. Available at: http://accessmedicine.mhmedical.com.online.uchc.edu/content.aspx?bookid=1130&Sectionid=79732627. Accessed August 30, 2015.
5. Jundt JP, Liem TK, Moneta GL. Venous and lymphatic disease. In: Brunicardi F, Andersen DK, Billiar TR, et al,

editors. Schwartz's principles of surgery. 10th edition. New York: McGraw-Hill; 2014. Available at: http://accesssurgery.mhmedical.com.online.uchc.edu/content.aspx?bookid=980&Sectionid=59610866. Accessed August 30, 2015.

6. Morimoto Y, Niwa H, Minematsu K. Risk factors affecting hemorrhage after tooth extraction in patients undergoing continuous infusion with unfractionated heparin. J Oral Maxillofac Surg 2012;70(3):521–6.

7. Lowry JC. Thromboembolic disease and thromboprophylaxis in oral and maxillofacial surgery: experience and practice. Br J Oral Maxillofac Surg 1995;33(?): 101–6.

8. Bajkin BV, Popovic SL, Selakovic SD. Randomized, prospective trial comparing bridging therapy using low-molecular-weight heparin with maintenance of oral anticoagulation during extraction of teeth. J Oral Maxillofac Surg 2009;67(5):990–5.

9. Farr DR, Hare AR. The use of thromboembolic prophylaxis in oral and maxillofacial surgery. Br J Oral Maxillofac Surg 1994;32(3):161–4.

Warfarin and Newer Agents
What the Oral Surgeon Needs to Know

Martin B. Steed, DDS*, Matthew T. Swanson, DDS

KEYWORDS

- Dabigatran • Rivaroxaban • Apixaban • Warfarin • Praxbind • Factor Xa inhibitors • Andexanet alfa

KEY POINTS

- Thromboprophylaxis with anticoagulants is an important aspect of managing patients at risk of systemic or pulmonary embolization.
- Dabigatran is a direct inhibitor of thrombin (Factor IIa).
- Rivaroxaban and apixaban inhibit Factor Xa.
- Monitoring of coagulation function is not routinely necessary with these new drugs but may be useful in emergencies.
- Praxbind in the only reversal agent approved by the US Food and Drug Administration for specific emergency situations.
- Nonspecific hemostatic agents that have been suggested for off-label use in reversing excessive bleeding in patients taking the new oral anticoagulants include recombinant Factor VIIa, 3-factor and 4-factor prothrombin complex concentrate, and activated prothrombin complex concentrate.

INTRODUCTION

The management of perioperative bleeding is a fundamental skill of the oral and maxillofacial surgeon that requires continual re-education as new medications become available for anticoagulation. In addition to vitamin K antagonists and heparins, anticoagulants that directly target the enzymatic activity of thrombin and Factor Xa have been developed. These are termed direct oral anticoagulants (DOACs).[1] Familiarity with the pharmacology of newer agents is essential for preoperative and postoperative management in order to safely treat anticoagulated patients.

The management of anticoagulation in patients undergoing surgical procedures is challenging, because interrupting anticoagulation for a procedure transiently increases the risk of thromboembolism. At the same time, surgery and invasive procedures have associated bleeding risks that are increased by the anticoagulants administered for venous thromboembolism prevention. If significant bleeding can be anticipated from the procedure (ie: free fibular osseomyocutaneous flap or coronal incision), their anticoagulant may need to be discontinued for a longer period, resulting in a longer period of increased thromboembolic risk. A personalized balance between reducing the risk of thromboembolism and preventing excessive bleeding must be reached for each patient.

Additional issues relate to the specific anticoagulant used. All anticoagulants increase bleeding risk. For those taking a vitamin K antagonist (eg, warfarin), it takes several days until the anticoagulant effect is reduced and then re-established

Disclosure Statement: The authors have nothing to disclose.
Department of Oral and Maxillofacial Surgery, Medical University of South Carolina, Room BSB 453 MSC 507, 173 Ashley Avenue, Charleston, SC 29425, USA
* Corresponding author.
E-mail address: steedma@musc.edu

Oral Maxillofacial Surg Clin N Am 28 (2016) 515–521
http://dx.doi.org/10.1016/j.coms.2016.06.011
1042-3699/16/© 2016 Elsevier Inc. All rights reserved.

perioperatively. The risks and benefits of bridging with a shorter-acting agent, such as heparin, during this time remain unclear. The newer direct oral anticoagulants (ie: direct thrombin inhibitor dabigatran, Factor Xa inhibitors rivaroxaban, apixaban, and edoxaban) have shorter half-lives, making them easier to discontinue and resume rapidly, but they lack a specific antidote or reversal strategy.[2] This raises concerns about treatment of bleeding and management of patients who require an urgent procedure as in the maxillofacial trauma patient. Interruption of anticoagulation temporarily increases thromboembolic risk, and continuing anticoagulation increases the risk of bleeding associated with invasive procedures; both of these outcomes adversely affect mortality. The approach to perioperative management of anticoagulation takes into account these risks, along with specific features of the anticoagulant the patient is taking.

Of note, many current approaches are based only at the evidential level of expert opinion.[3,4] Thrombotic and bleeding risks may vary depending on individual circumstances, and data from randomized trials are not available to guide practice in many settings. In addition, the best surrogate for complete resolution of anticoagulant effect is not always known or available for the newer target-specific anticoagulants. Thus, this approach should be used as a guideline and should not substitute for clinician judgment in decisions about perioperative anticoagulant management.

An approach to decision making is outlined in this article.

ESTIMATE THROMBOEMBOLIC RISK

A higher thromboembolic risk increases the importance of minimizing the interval without anticoagulation. Thromboembolic risk for patients with atrial fibrillation is estimated based on age and comorbidities. For those with a recent deep vein thrombosis or pulmonary embolism, the risk is estimated based on the interval since diagnosis. If thromboembolic risk is transiently increased (ie, recent stroke or pulmonary embolism), surgeons should delay surgery until the risk returns to baseline, if possible. For patients with more than 1 condition that predisposes to thromboembolism, the condition with the highest thromboembolic risk takes precedence.

ESTIMATE BLEEDING RISK

A higher bleeding risk confers a greater need for perioperative hemostasis, and hence a longer period of anticoagulant interruption. Bleeding risk is dominated by the type and urgency of surgery; some patient comorbidities also contribute. Procedures with a low bleeding risk (ie: dental extractions or minor skin surgery) often can be performed without interruption of anticoagulation.

DETERMINE THE TIMING OF ANTICOAGULANT INTERRUPTION

The timing of anticoagulant interruption depends on the specific agent the patient is receiving. For example, warfarin requires earlier discontinuation than the shorter-acting target-specific oral anticoagulants (ie: dabigatran, rivaroxaban, apixaban) (Table 1).

DETERMINE WHETHER TO USE BRIDGING ANTICOAGULATION

For patients receiving warfarin, the interval without an anticoagulant may be as long as 5 to 6 days due to the long half-life of warfarin and time to reach the therapeutic international normalized ratio (INR) range. The use of heparin or low molecular weight heparin (LMWH) to reduce the interval without anticoagulation (ie, bridging anticoagulation) may be appropriate for some patients, especially those who have a high thromboembolic risk.

DIRECT ORAL ANTICOAGULANTS
Xa Inhibitors

Direct Factor Xa inhibitors are a new class of anticoagulation medications that are increasingly being substituted for vitamin K antagonists and LMWH for appropriate patients (Fig. 1). The xabans (Xa ban = inhibitor) include rivaroxaban, apixaban, edoxaban, and Betrixaban (in development) act directly on Factor Xa in the coagulation cascade and are gaining popularity due to the need for less monitoring, fairly quick onset and offset of action, few drug interactions, and no food interactions, which provide a greater convenience to patients and a more consistent therapeutic blood level.

IIa Inhibitors

Direct thrombin inhibitors, dabigatran, bivalirudin, argatroban, desirudin, are similar to the Xa inhibitors, but target Factor IIa and cause direct inhibition of thrombin. These too have few drug interactions and no food interactions, making them a popular alternative to warfarin.

MECHANISM OF ACTION

Direct Factor Xa inhibitors work by preventing Factor Xa from cleaving prothrombin to thrombin.

Table 1
Profiles of warfarin and the newer direct oral anticoagulants

	Warfarin	Dabigatran	Rivaroxaban	Apixaban
Mechanism of action	Vitamin K antagonist (Factors II, VII, IX, X)	Direct thrombin inhibitor (Factor II)	Factor Xa inhibitor	Factor Xa inhibitor
Reversal	*Rapid:* FFP and vitamin K 1–5 mg *Delayed:* Vitamin K 1–5 mg PO	PraxBind 5 g	4-factor prothrombin complex concentrate 50 units/kg 3-factor with FFP Activated prothrombin complex concentrate 50–100 units/kg	4-factor prothrombin complex concentrate 50 units/kg 3-factor with FFP Activated prothrombin complex concentrate 50–100 units/kg
Monitoring	INR	Ecarin clotting time aPTT	Anti-Xa	Anti-Xa
Surgical concerns	INR <3.0 Local hemostatic measures	Wait 24–48 h Local hemostatic measures	Wait 24–48 h Local hemostatic measures	Wait 24–48 h Local hemostatic measures

The formation of a stable clot is the result of a complex interaction between multiple coagulation factors. The coagulation cascade begins through 2 initial pathways, the contact activation pathway, also referred to as the intrinsic pathway, and the tissue factor pathway, also known as the extrinsic pathway, that lead to a common pathway resulting in fibrin formation. Most coagulation factors are enzymes (serine proteases) that act by cleaving downstream proteins and combine at Factor Xa, which is the common factor and gateway to thrombin activation and the formation of a fibrin clot. Direct Factor Xa inhibitors work immediately upstream of thrombin formation by directly inactivating the circulating and clot-bound factor Xa through binding to the active site of factor Xa.

One advantage of direct factor Xa inhibitors is their ability to block both forms of Xa; additionally, they do not require a cofactor, whereas indirect inhibitors such as heparin only inactive the fluid phase of Xa. The majority of the Factor Xa inhibitor is metabolized in the liver, and approximately 25% to 35% of Factor Xa is metabolized in the kidney; therefore, hepatic insufficiency could lead to accumulation.

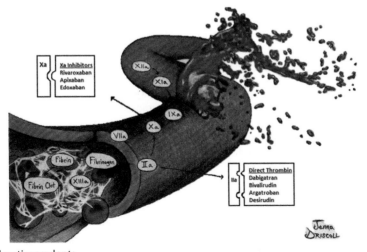

Fig. 1. Direct oral anticoagulants.

Direct thrombin inhibitors, such as dabigatran, inactivate clot-bound and circulating thrombin, which is the final enzyme that cleaves fibrinogen to fibrin, as well as activating Factors V, VIII, XI, XIII and platelets.

MONITORING

Routine coagulation tooling is not used for determining the anticoagulation status of a patient receiving a DOAC. Prolonged coagulation times can be helpful in determining residual effect, but normal results cannot necessarily prove that the anticoagulant effect has resolved.[1] The primary monitor of the xabans is the measurement of anti-Xa activity, which is a plasma assay performed through a chromogenic procedure. A sample of the patient's plasma is added to a known amount of Factor Xa, which leads to a binding with the Factor Xa inhibitor. The amount of residual factor Xa is inversely proportional to the amount of Factor Xa inhibitor, which is detected by adding a substrate that when cleaved releases a chromophore that is detected by a spectrophotometer. The quantity of chromophore released is inversely proportional to the Factor Xa inhibitor, and each chromophore released is measured against a calibration curve.

The primary monitor of the direct thrombin inhibitors, like dabigatran, is the activated partial thromboplastin time (aPTT). Patients who are anticoagulated will have an elevated aPTT, above the normal range of 30 to 50 seconds. Another measurement tool, the ecarin clotting time (ECT) is becoming more available to determine direct thrombin inhibitor levels. A known quantity of ecarin is added to the patient's plasma, and the ECT is prolonged in a linear relationship to the plasma level of direct thrombin inhibitor. A chromogenic substrate can also be added to the sample to provide an ecarin chromogenic assay.

Factor Xa and direct thrombin inhibitors are becoming a popular alternative to warfarin due to the fact they do not require frequent monitoring. Unlike warfarin, which has a number of medication and food interactions, Xa inhibitors maintain a more consistent therapeutic level. For the simple, outpatient oral surgical procedures, routine Factor Xa level monitoring may not be necessary, and local hemostatic measures may suffice. However, in the trauma and high-risk surgical risk patient, knowing the level of anticoagulation may be prudent.

BLEEDING RISK FROM DIRECT ORAL ANTICOAGULANTS

Risks of bleeding form DOACs are generally lower than or similar to other agents.

Outcomes of DOAC-associated bleeding appear favorable compared with vitamin k antagonists as demonstrated by a 2015 meta-analysis that included 13 randomized clinical trials in over 100,000 patients.[5] Severity of bleeding and degree of anticoagulation were assessed by patient history and physical examination. The degree of anticoagulation depended on the dose and the interval since the last dose.

REVERSAL

Andexanet alfa is the only specific factor Xa antidote for use as a reversal agent for those patients taking rivaroxaban and apixaban. As the use of Factor Xa anticoagulants becomes more prevalent in the general population, the need for a specific reversal agent becomes more urgent. It is estimated that from April 2014 to 2015, there were more than 50,000 patients admitted for Factor Xa inhibitor-related bleedings, and the number is expected to continually rise. Portola Pharmaceuticals (San Francisco, California) published Phase 3 studies in the *New England Journal of Medicine* in November 2015 and have received US Food and Drug Administration (FDA) approval for use in life-threatening and uncontrolled bleeding.[6] Andexanet alfa is a catalytically inactive recombinant human protein that binds with high affinity to Factor Xa inhibitors within the bloodstream, thereby increasing effective Factor Xa levels and decreasing overall anticoagulation.

Prior to the development of Andexanet, the primary reversal for those patients at imminent risk of death from bleeding due to direct Factor Xa anticoagulation was inactivated 4-factor prothrombin complex concentrates (PCC) at 50 units/kg or 3-factor PCC with fresh-frozen plasma. Clinical evidence to support this practice is not available, and clinical judgment is necessary on a case-by-case basis. Recombinant Factor VIIa administration has shown efficacy for reversal of anti-Xa medications in minor bleeds. but further research is needed for guidelines in major bleeds. For those patients with a major bleed, antifibrinolytic agents such as tranexamic acid or e-aminocaproic acid can be administered. Dialysis is a not an effective tool, because the inhibitors are highly protein-bound and charcoal hemofiltration has not been fully evaluated. Those patients with minor bleeding can be managed with local conservative measures.

Direct thrombin inhibitors are the only newer agents that have an FDA-approved specific reversal agent, idarucizumab. On October 16, 2015 the FDA granted accelerated approval for use in patients during emergency situations/urgent procedures for life-threatening or uncontrolled bleeding. The medication is a humanized monoclonal antibody fragment that binds to dabigatran and its metabolites with a higher affinity than dabigatran to thrombin, thereby neutralizing the anticoagulation effects. It comes supplied as 2 separate vials of 2.5 g/50 mL and has a recommended dose of 5 g, there are limited data to support additional dosages. The reported adverse effects of this medication are headache (>5%), hypokalemia, delirium, constipation, pyrexia, and pneumonia (<5%). Activated prothrombin complex concentrate administration has been used to reverse dabigatran in life-threatening bleeds, but further research is needed to support its use. Patients on direct thrombin inhibitors who are at risk with a major bleed should be managed with appropriate hemodynamic support and can undergo hemodialysis and/or activated charcoal, administration of antifibrinolytic agents, and clotting factor products.

WARFARIN

Since 1954, the vitamin K antagonist warfarin has been a popular medication for anticoagulation to prevent deep vein thrombosis and thromboembolism in at-risk patients. First developed as a pesticide to combat rats and mice, it has become the workhorse for anticoagulation in the worldwide population. It is estimated that 2 million people take warfarin every year, and it is the second most common drug behind insulin involved in emergency room visits for adverse drug events. In the United States, it is the most commonly prescribed oral anticoagulant. Warfarin works by inhibiting the vitamin K-dependent clotting Factors II, VII, IX, X by binding to epoxide reductase, thereby reducing the available vitamin K. In addition to clotting factors, it also effects the coagulation regulatory factors protein C, protein S, and protein Z. Although it is widely prescribed and affordable to patients, it has several limitations because of its food and drug interactions. Those foods with high vitamin K content (ie, leaf vegetables and greens) affect the anticoagulation levels of warfarin. Many antibiotics commonly used in the oral and maxillofacial surgery field can alter the efficacy of warfarin. For example, amoxicillin, amoxicillin-clavulanate, ciprofloxacin, levofloxacin, metronidazole, and sulfamethoxazole may increase the anticoagulation effect of warfarin. Other antibiotics, like dicloxacillin, nafcillin, rifampin, and rifapentine may decrease the anticoagulant activity of warfarin. Due to the many food and drug interactions, warfarin requires frequent, routine monitoring through the international normalized ratio (INR).

MONITORING AND REVERSAL

Warfarin levels are monitored by the INR, which is a calculation of the patient's prothrombin time compared with a control sample. Prothrombin time is a measurement of the plasma time to clot after addition of tissue factor, measuring the

Table 2
Warfarin dosing recommendations

Procedures	Examples	INR Level	Coumadin Dosing
Low risk	• Single extraction • Soft tissue biopsy/excision of soft tissue lesion ≤1 cm in diameter	• <3.5 • Local hemostatic measures	• No change • Local hemostatic measures
Medium risk	• Multiple extractions: ≤5 teeth • Soft tissue biopsy/excision of soft tissue lesion 1–3 cm in diameter • Placement of 1–3 dental implants	• <3.0 • Local hemostatic measures	• Withhold 1–2 d prior[a] • Restart within 24 h
High risk	• Multiple extractions >5 teeth or surgical • Open mandible fracture repair • Soft tissue biopsy/excision of soft tissue lesion >3 cm • Biopsy/excision of a hard tissue lesion • Removal of maxillary and/or mandibular tori • Placement of multiple dental implants: >3 implants	• <2.5 • Local hemostatic measures	• Withhold 2–4 d • Restart within 24 h

[a] Recommend consultation with prescribing physician.

Table 3
Vitamin K administration to reverse elevated international normalized ratios

INR Value	Urgent OMFS Surgery	OMFS Surgery in 24–28 h
INR $\geq$1.0 but $\leq$3.0	Local hemostatic measures Treatment with FFP	Vitamin K 1 mg PO
INR >3.0 but $\leq$5	For rapid (<12 h) reversal: FFP + vitamin K 1–3 mg slowly intravenously	Vitamin K 1–2.5 mg PO Repeat every 24 h as needed for appropriate INR
INR >5 but <9	For rapid (<12 h) reversal: FFP + vitamin K 2–5 mg slowly intravenously	Vitamin K 2.5–5 mg orally Repeat every 24 h as needed for appropriate INR Vitamin K 1–2 mg orally

extrinsic pathway of coagulation. The INR is necessary for monitoring warfarin, because a patient's anticoagulation level can fluctuate greatly. Each patient is tailored to a specific regimen; however, diet, personal factors (eg, missing dosages), and the short half-life of Factor VII at 3 to 6 hours can cause large changes in INR level. Warfarin interacts with the vitamin K-dependent factors; therefore a diet high in greens like salad greens, leafy vegetables, lettuce, and spinach will lower the effective INR. For those patients at a low risk of thromboembolism, the American College of Chest Physicians recommends withholding warfarin 4 to 5 days preoperatively (**Table 2**).[7]

The usual therapeutic target range for anticoagulation is 2.0 to 3.0 but depends on the medical condition and the specific patient (ie, those with mechanical heart valves typically have a higher INR goal). Procedures with a low bleeding risk (eg, dental extractions and minor skin surgery) can typically be performed with an INR below 3.0 and do not require reversal of warfarin. Ideally, a patient will have an INR level checked the day of surgery or within 24 hours. However, depending on the patient's compliance and previous INR levels, it is the surgeon's preference to proceed with a recent INR within the past few days. If any doubt should arise, it is always prudent to obtain a new, current INR. After most outpatient oral surgery procedures, warfarin should be restarted within 24 hours at the usual dose.

In emergency situations and life threatening hemorrhage, FFP is administered to reverse elevated INRs, typically an initial dose of 2 to 4 units. Vitamin K can also be administered either orally or intravenously and simultaneously with FFP for rapid reversal of elevated INRs (**Table 3**). However, this reversal treatment does not come without its complications and puts patients at risk to develop deep vein thrombosis, pulmonary embolism, and ischemic stroke. The *Annals of Emergency Medicine* reported thrombotic events at 7.3% in patients receiving 4-factor prothrombin complex concentrate and 7.1% in those receiving plasma out of 2 randomized studies involving 388 patients.[8]

SUMMARY

Many oral and maxillofacial surgical patients have hematological disorders that interfere with a proper clot formation or take medications to alter their coagulation status and place them at an increased risk for postoperative hemorrhage. Patients with atrial fibrillation, previous strokes, deep vein thrombosis, myocardial infarction or pulmonary embolism have historically been treated with vitamin K inhibitors like warfarin, which required frequent monitoring and a stable diet. With new pharmacologic advances, many patients are now being treated with direct Factor Xa inhibitors, a new drug classification that is showing clinical promise as a substitute for warfarin and offers many advantages including less frequent monitoring and no food interactions. Although long-term data are unavailable because of their limited prospective experience, Factor Xa inhibitors have the potential to become the mainstay of pharmacologic anticoagulation.

Direct oral anticoagulants reversibly inhibit their target and have a shorter half-life than warfarin. Decisions to temporarily discontinue the DOAC must balance the bleeding and thrombotic risk for each patient. In cases in which there already is DOAC contributory bleeding, the drug is discontinued; the anatomic region is addressed primarily (pressure, surgery, local measures), and the patient is transfused blood products as needed. Additionally, antifibrinolytics are administered.

REFERENCES

1. Barnes GD, Ageno W, Ansell J, et al. Recommendation on the nomenclature for oral anticoagulants: communication from the SSC of the ISTH. J Thromb Haemost 2015;13:1154.

2. Garcia DA, Crowther M. Management of bleeding in patients receiving direct oral anticoagulants. In: Tirnhauer JS, editor. UpToDate. Available at: http://www.uptodate.com/home. Accessed February 15, 2016.

3. Siegal DM, Garcia DA, Crowther MA. How I treat target-specific oral anticoagulant bleeding. Blood 2014;123:1152.

4. Kaatz S, Koudes PA, Garcia DA, et al. Guidance on the emergent reversal of oral thrombin and factor Xa inhibitors. Am J Hematol 2012;87(Suppl 1):S141.

5. Chai-Adisaksopha C, Hillis C, Isayama T, et al. Mortality outcomes in patients receiving direct oral anticoagulants: a systematic review and meta-analysis of randomized controlled trials. J Thromb Haemost 2012;2015:13.

6. Siegal DM, Curnutte JT, Connolly SJ, et al. Andexanet Alfa for the reversal of factor Xa inhibitor activity. N Engl J Med 2015;373:2413–24.

7. Daley BJ, et al. Perioperative anticoagulation management. Medscape. Available at: http://emedicine.medscape.com/article/285265-overview. Accessed March 7, 2016.

8. Milling TJ, Refaai MA, Goldstein JN, et al. Thromboembolic events after vitamin K antagonist reversal with 4-factor prothrombin complex concentrate: analyses of two randomized, plasma-controlled studies. Ann Emerg Med 2016;67(1):96–105.

Topical Hemostatic Agents
What the Oral and Maxillofacial Surgeon Needs to Know

Patrick J. Vezeau, DDS, MS

KEYWORDS

- Topical hemostatic agents • Hemostasis • Oral and maxillofacial surgery

KEY POINTS

- Hemostatic agents can be useful adjuncts for oral and maxillofacial surgery procedures.
- Knowledge of normal and abnormal hemostatic mechanisms is necessary to safely practice surgery.
- Different hemostatic agents can be used, depending on the type of surgery and estimated or actual blood loss encountered.
- Cost factors must be weighed against efficacy and side-effect profiles when selecting a topical hemostatic agent.

INTRODUCTION

Hemostasis is a key concept in the safe practice of any surgical procedure. This concept is especially true for any procedures of the head and neck, where the local robust vascular supply exists with the necessity of maintenance of a patent airway. Loss of hemostasis after dentoalveolar procedures has been documented to compromise the airway and cause hypovolemia, even in otherwise healthy individuals without known bleeding diatheses.[1] Orthognathic surgery usually carries a greater risk of significant blood loss, generally increasing with the number of surgical sites/procedures.[2,3] Major head and neck procedures to address neoplasia may further increase both blood loss and the probable need for transfusion of bank blood products.[4] Therefore, concentration on prevention of blood loss in surgery is a laudable goal. Herein is presented a review of various methods of topical hemostasis with which oral and maxillofacial surgeons may wish to take advantage.

REVIEW OF NORMAL HEMOSTASIS

Although a complex process, hemostasis can be divided into 4 distinct phases[5]:

1. Vascular contraction—acutely injured arteries and arterioles, having a muscular tunica media, are able to undergo vasospasm to decrease the amount of intravascular fluid loss.
2. Endothelial injury and platelet plug formation—endothelial cell injury and subendothelial collagen exposure causes adhesion of platelets under the influence of von Willebrand factor. Aggregation of other platelets is followed by conformational changes in platelets and liberation of several substances that increase both platelet aggregation and direct activation of thrombin.
3. Initiation of the clotting cascade—this has classically been described as having 2 arms, the extrinsic (tissue factor activated) and the intrinsic (intravascular) pathways, which join at the common pathway. At that stage, activated

Private Practice, 301 Oak Tree Lane, Dakota Dunes, SD 57049, USA
E-mail address: pjvezeau@oralsurgery-implants.com

Oral Maxillofacial Surg Clin N Am 28 (2016) 523–532
http://dx.doi.org/10.1016/j.coms.2016.06.007
1042-3699/16/$ – see front matter © 2016 Elsevier Inc. All rights reserved.

factor X complex cleaves prothombin to thrombin, forming a complex that then cleaves fibrinogen to fibrin, which then forms a network of cross-linked fibrin mesh that ensnares the platelets and erythrocytes to form a retracted clot. The details of this cascade have recently been found to be much more interactive and complex than originally thought, with multiple positive and negative feedback mechanisms.[6]

4. Modulation of clotting—plasma antithrombin and tissue factor pathway inhibitor, which freely circulate, are negative amplifiers of the coagulation cascade. Proteins C and S are activated by several proteins in the coagulation pathway, inhibiting activated factors V and VII. As a part of healing, several proteolytic enzymes, notably plasmin (activated by tissue plasminogen activator or urokinase), disrupt the fibrin clot into fibrin degradation products, restoring blood vessel patency.

BLEEDING DIATHESIS

Blood loss associated with surgery can be magnified by the presence of a bleeding diathesis. Such a state may be acquired, autoimmune, or genetic and may involve either the formation of the platelet plug, coagulation pathway, or both[7] (**Box 1**). Such situations may make the use of appropriate topical hemostatic agents desirable.

OVERVIEW OF TOPICAL HEMOSTATIC AGENTS

Certain surgical procedures (vascular procedures, nerves grafts, and large open surgical defects of soft tissue) do not lend themselves to physical methods of hemostasis, such as electrocautery or chemical cautery. Other patients have bleeding disorders that may not be totally correctable prior to surgery and can benefit from the use of topical hemostatic agents. Topical agents are not to be used intravascularly or unintended thrombosis can occur.

Topical hemostatic agents can be classified as scaffold/matrix, biologically active, styptic, tissue adhesive, sealant, occlusive, and vasoconstrictive. Each has indications for application, drawbacks, and contraindications, which are reviewed.

Scaffold/Matrix Agents

Scaffold/matrix agents have been available for decades and are widely used in all areas of surgery. They are generally applied as a dry agent and allowed to help propagate the fibrin/platelet matrix. Four types of agents are generally available:

> **Box 1**
> **Summary of hemorrhagic diatheses**
>
> *Disorders of platelets*
>
> Thrombocytopenias
>
>   Immune thrombocytopenias
>
>   Drug-induced thrombocytopenias (chemotherapy and heparin-induced)
>
>   Myelodysplasia/aplastic anemia
>
>   Hypersplenism
>
> Alterations in platelet function
>
>   Adhesion disorders (genetic)
>
>   von Willebrand disease
>
>   Therapeutic platelet inhibitors
>
> $P2Y_{12}$ inhibitors (clopidrogel and prasugrel)
>
>   Cyclo-oxygenase inhibitors (aspirin)
>
>   Phosphidiesterase inhibitors (cilostazol)
>
>   GP IIB/IIIA inhibitors
>
>   Adenosine reuptake inhibitors (persantine)
>
> *Disorders of coagulation*
>
> Hemophilias
>
>   Factor VII (classic/A), IX (B), and XI (C), others
>
>   Liver dysfunction
>
>   Factor antibody syndromes
>
> Therapeutic anticoagulants
>
>   Warfarin
>
>   Heparins
>
>   Factor X inhibitors (rivaroxaban and apixaban)
>
>   Factor II inhibitor (dabigatran)
>
> Diffuse intravascular coagulopathy
>
> Massive transfusion states

---

gelatin matrix, microfibrillar collagen, porous polysaccharides, and oxidized methylcellulose.

Gelatin matrix

Processed from porcine dermal collagen product that is fomented and dried, gelatin matrix has a neutral pH. Marketed as Gelfoam (Pfizer, New York, NY) and Surgifoam (Ethicon US LLC, Somerville, NJ), gelatin matrix is available as a sponge or as a powder.[8] It is believed to provide a porous matrix in which platelet enmeshing and fibrin clot formation are supported. Extremely hygroscopic, gelatin matrix can absorb 40 times its weight in fluid.[9] Doing so, it increases in size and may cause surrounding wound pressure, furthering hemostasis. Gelatin matrix is resorbed by hydrolysis in 4 to 6 weeks. Increased incidences of infection and granuloma formation have been reported.[10] Although technically a xenograft, little allergic activity has been reported with gelatin matrix products.

Microfibrillar collagen
Microfibrillar collagen is produced from bovine collagen and acts by causing platelet adherence and activation, thus initiating formation of a platelet plug and a subsequent fibrin mesh network.[11] It is available as a powder (Avitene, Bard Davol, Warwick, RI) which can be compressed into nonwoven sheets. More limited hemostasis can be expected in cases of thrombocytopenia. Microfibrillar powder or sheet collagen does not significantly swell when exposed to fluids. Proteolytic resorption is accomplished in approximately 8 weeks. One study showed significantly shorted hemostasis time when compared with oxidized methylcellulose.[12] This product can pass through blood filters and should not be used with surgical blood recycling. Microfibrillar collagen has been processed into plugs (CollaPlug, Zimmer, Warsaw, IN) and sheets (CollaTape, Zimmer, Warsaw, IN) to achieve hemostasis in extraction sites and graft sites, respectively,[13] as well as for other oral surgical grafting procedures.

Oxidized cellulose
Produced from wood pulp cellulose, oxidized cellulose is a chain of loosely connected cellulose chains. It readily conforms to surgical sites and does not adhere to surgical instruments.[14] Available in sheets (Surgicel, Ethicon US LLC, Somerville, NJ), oxidized cellulose has an acidic pH, causing red cell lysis and formation of a pseudoclot. Theoretically, this low pH may also be antimicrobial.[15] Use of other hemostatic agents, such as topical thrombin (discussed later), is not possible in such an acidic environment. Although small amounts are absorbed in approximately 8 weeks, larger amounts take longer. Additionally, the acidic pH may delay resorption and cause postsurgical adhesions and other complications.[16,17]

Microporous mucopolysaccharide spheres
Microporous mucopolysaccharide spheres (Arista AH, Bard Davol, Warwick, RI) are processed from potato starch and processed into microporous spheres, which are applied topically to the surgical site after initial drying with a sponge. The pore size acts as water sieve and dehydrates the surgical field, concentrating erythrocytes and platelets, aiding in hemostasis. These are resorbed in 24 to 48 hours by tissue amylases and are nonpyogenic.

These have been used with favorable results in several surgical applications with a good safety record.[18,19] A lower efficacy of topical hemostasis, however, compared with procoagulant hemostatic matrix materials has been reported.[20]

Biological Hemostats

Biologically active hemostatic agents include procoagulant medications (thrombin) or antifibrinolytics (epsilon-aminocaproic acid [EACA] and tranexamic acid [TA]). Additionally, naturally occurring procoagulant substances are commonly used as topical hemostatics.

Topical thrombin
Topical use of factor II (thrombin) initiates the cleavage of fibrinogen to fibrin, forming a fibrin clot. Originally commercially available as a derivative of bovine plasma, troublesome immunologic reactions have been common with this preparation.[21] This led to the use of pooled human plasma thrombin, which had concern with infectious disease transmission. More recently, recombinant human thrombin preparations have become common and avoid the previously stated issues.[22] Reconstituted from a lyophilized powder, thrombin liquid can be applied topically (often with a sprayer), usually with several minutes of pressure by a damp sponge.

Antifibrinolytics
Lysis of the fibrin clot occurs by plasmin activity. Antifibrinolytics, such as EACA and TA, are synthetically derived analogs of the amino acid lysine and bind to the lysine-binding sites on plasmin, thereby preventing proteolysis of the fibrin clot.[23] Either medication can be used topically or systemically. TA is approximately 10 times more potent than EACA[24] and most studies of topical antifibrinolytics have involved TA. Perioperative TA oral rinses (approximately 5% solutions) starting immediately preoperatively and continuing every 6 hours for 7 days have been found beneficial in patients with hemophilia A[25] and warfarin anticoagulation.[26,27] Perioperative TA mouthwash use has received expert recommendation for invasive dental treatment of patients on oral antithrombotic medications.[28] A small sample size study of bimaxillary orthognathic surgery demonstrated statistically significant reduction of intraoperative blood loss with the use of a 1% TA irrigating solution in saline versus saline placebo.[29]

Naturally occurring procoagulants
Hemocoagulase Hemocoagulase is a pharmacologic preparation of coagulative proteins extracted from the venom of *Bothrops jararaca* or *Bothrops*

atrox. These proteases cleave fibrinogen to fibrin and also act as a factor X activator. The formed fibrin mesh is formed independently of thrombin activity and is, therefore, resistant to plasma antithrombin and is not dependent on serum calcium for activation.[28] Studies have demonstrated that topical application of hemocoagulase significantly decreases postextraction bleeding and edema when compared with controls.[30,31] Although used in South Asia and Japan, hemocoagulase has not yet received Food and Drug Administration approval.

Chitin/chitosan dressings Chitin is a naturally occurring polysaccharide found both in arthropod exoskeletons and as a fermentation product of algae, whereas chitosan is its deacylated form. Both forms are believed to promote hemostasis by local vasoconstriction and by acting as a scaffold for erythrocyte agglutination. These topical dressings also physically occlude the bleeding surgical site and possess antimicrobial properties due to having an acidic pH.[32] These materials stimulate fibroblast activation and collagen deposition. A topical form for emergency field trauma (HemeCon, Tricol Biomedical, Portland, OR) is supplied as a flat bandage with chitosan on one side (to be applied to the wound) and a nonstick side facing away from the wound to allow topical pressure to be applied. Chitosan dressings are currently used in both military field medical and civilian emergency medical service settings and show promise as possible guided tissue scaffolds.[33]

Mineral zeolite Derived for kaolin (powdered oxides of Al, Na, Si, Mg, Na, and other cations), these topical dressings cause local dehydration and concentration of erythrocytes and platelets as well as directly activating factor XII to initiate the coagulation cascade.[34] A commercial form (QuickClot, Z-Medica LLC, Wallingford, CT) is used for external application and now is supplied as the partially hydrated zeolite powder on a gauze mesh (QuickClot ACS Sponge) to allow external pressure to be applied to the wound and decrease exothermic properties of the dehydrated zeolite product.[35] This material cannot be left in place during wound closure as a foreign body reaction and/or infection may ensue. This material is stable and cost-effective.

Alginate dressings Calcium or zinc alginate dressings may be applied to topical wounds for hemostasis via tissue fluid absorption and concentration of cellular blood components as well as cationic initiation of the coagulation cascade[36] and providing a barrier. These are most often used to dress cutaneous exudative wounds because they can be removed with water only with minimal disruption of underlying healing tissues.[37] They are not, however, effective situations involving a high flow of blood.

Styptics

Styptic agents arrest hemorrhage by their astringent properties (ie, causing tissue and blood vessel contraction by chemical or osmotic means). A common type of dermatologic hemostyptic is an anhydrous aluminum salt styptic pencil (discussed later). In intraoral surgical procedures, povidone-iodine preparations applied topically to tissue beds have been shown to have styptic and anti-infective properties when used in periapical surgery.[38]

Hydrophilic polymers with potassium salts

Used in topical dermatologic situations, the over-the-counter preparations, hydrophilic polymers with potassium salts, are powders including a hydrophilic micropolymer particulate combined with potassium ferrate[39] (BioSeal and WoundSeal, Biolife, Sarasota, FL). The polymer causes initial dehydration and the potassium salt acts as a binding agent, causing aggregation of erythrocytes and platelets. The end product is an artificial eschar that exfoliates after healing of underlying tissues. Reasonably good efficacy has been demonstrated in dermatologic surgical sites.[40] Hydrophilic polymers with potassium salts cannot, however, be used in wounds that will be closed because the micropolymer portion is not resorbed.

Mineral salts

Mineral salts are commonly used as a topical application for localized dermal bleeding. These can be used in the form of a pencil or solutions to be topically applied. Mineral salts cause coagulation of proteins, tissue necrosis, and contraction and ensuing vascular thrombus formation.[41] Commonly used salts include silver nitrate, aluminum chloride, zinc salts, and ferric sulfate (as Monsel solution). Both silver and iron salts[42] are effective local hemostats. Although these possess anti-infective properties, permanent dermal pigmentation from liberal use of iron and silver salts has been reported.[43] If used on cutaneous bleeding surfaces, frequent gentle wiping with a damp saline soaked gauze may help minimize this discoloration. Zinc chloride applied as a topical paste (often prepackaged on gauze squares) has a long history of use in Mohs surgery.[44] Although its fixative properties have been useful in this application, delayed healing and pain have caused it to be supplanted by other available agents.[45]

Various salts of aluminum (most often aluminum chloride) are commonly used in dermatology due to lack of pigmentation with their use. These can be directly applied as a solid topically or as a solution (20%–40%). Compared with other mineral salts, aluminum does not cause tissue discoloration, leading to its common use in contemporary dermatologic surgery. Delayed healing with over-vigorous use, however, has been reported as a complication.[46]

Tissue Sealants

Tissue sealants combine biologically active agents (such as thrombin and fibrinogen) to form a hemostatic sealant[47] (Tisseel, Baxter, Deerfield, IL). Fibrin sealants are 2 component systems that use pooled or recombinant human thrombin/calcium with cryoprecipitate human fibrinogen. When using the supplied applicator, the 2 components are mixed on application, forming a fibrin clot seal. Although excellent topical hemostasis has been shown in general surgery applications, disease transmissibility is a concern. In some products TA is added as an antifibrinolytic. FloSeal (Baxter, Deerfield, IL) combines a bovine-derived microgranular gelatin flowable matrix (which swells and acts as a tamponading agent) with thrombin but no fibrinogen, so fibrin clotting requires exposure to a patient's native fibrinogen (ie, exposure to patient blood). Autologous plasma can be used as a fibrin source with recombinant thrombin, either with a platelet-poor or platelet-rich plasma technique.[48,49] This technique requires centrifugation of a sample of the patient's blood. In addition to increased hemostasis from platelet action, this technique causes concentration of platelet factors, which have been noted to have beneficial effects on bone and soft tissue healing.[50,51]

Tissue Adhesives

Tissue adhesives are used for tissue closure and approximation. The physical approximation of tissues can help in tamponade of bleeding. These adhesives can be tissue resorbed or nonresorbable.

Cyanoacrylates are liquid acrylate monomers that polymerize when exposed to tissue fluids. Two types are available: those with shorter side chains (Histoacryl, B Braun USA, Bethlehem, PA) or longer side chains (Dermabond and Surgiseal). Shorter side-chain adhesives cure more quickly and are stronger but more brittle with a higher likelihood of dehiscence.[52] Longer side-chained substances take longer to set but are more flexible.[53] Either are sloughed off during healing. If closed over, however, entrapped cyanoacrylate is broken down to cyanoacetate and formaldehyde, which can cause tissue toxicity and inflammatory reactions. By their nature, cyanoacrylates lend themselves to use in closure of cutaneous incisions and lacerations in situations where minimal tension exists or support has been gained by close approximation in deeper layers.

Polyethylene glycol hydrogel is a 2-phase application combining 2 forms of polyethylene glycol that, when applied topically, form a hydrogel matrix (Coseal, Baxter). This has been used as a topical hemostatic agent in vascular and urologic surgery[54] and has been found effective in repair of cerebrospinal fluid leak.[55] This material does swell, however, to at least 4 times its original size and should not be used in applications where this would compromise surgical site tissues.

Albumin-based–bovine-derived albumin can be cross-linked by gluteraldehyde (BioGlue). A 2-cartridge applicator mixes and applies this material topically, forming a tough, adhesive, and hemostatic matrix scaffold and is often used as an adjunct sealant in major vascular repairs. The adhesive properties have been used in endoscopic brow lift procedures.[56] As with any bovine-derived substance, however, prion transmission and hypersensitivity remain a theoretic risk.

Occlusive Agents

Bone wax

The occlusive agent, bone wax, is commonly used for osseous bleeding. A mixture of beeswax, paraffin, and softening agents, bone wax is inexpensive and has a long history of surgical use for medullary bone bleeding. This substance is nonabsorbable, however, and can impair bone healing, cause granuloma formation,[57] and act as a nidus of infection.[58] If used, the minimal amount to gain hemostasis should be used with removal of excess amounts.

Alkylene oxide copolymer

A biocompatable product with physical handling and occlusive properties similar to bone wax is Ostene (Baxter). This substance is an alkylene oxide copolymer material that is hydrophilic and water soluble.[59] Although causing occlusion of medullary vascular channels to obtain hemostasis, this material does not elicit a foreign body granuloma reaction and its removal over several weeks prevents it from acting as an infective nidus.[60] Advocates favor its use to replace bone wax in most osseous surgical procedures.

Vasoconstrictors and Epinephrine

The α_1 peripheral vasoconstricting qualities of epinephrine have long been valued in local hemostasis. Caution must be exercised when injecting large quantities of even dilute (1:200,000–500,000) solutions in patients with cardiovascular compromise or who may be taking nonselective β-blockers to avoid an unopposed α_1 hypertensive episode.[61] Previous recommendations that epinephrine be avoided in procedures involving the nose, ear lobes, fingers, or toes have recently been contradicted by studies showing that lower concentration epinephrine solutions (1:200,000) show no evidence of ischemia or necrosis when used judiciously.[62] Tumescent techniques using extremely dilute local anesthetic/vasoconstrictor solutions (such as lidocaine 0.1% with epinephrine 1:1,000,000) have been extensively used to minimize blood loss in liposuction[63] and maxillofacial cosmetic[64,65] procedures, producing hemostasis by vasoconstriction and by pneumatic occlusion of local vasculature.

Electrical and Laser Hemostasis

Applied electricity and laser energy to tissue for both surgery and hemostasis have been used for decades. Surgeons using these modalities, however, must keep in mind not only the physics and the desired goal but also contraindications and complications when applying energy directly to tissue.

Electrosurgery and electrocautery

Electrocautery Electrocautery uses heat generated by a passing an alternating or direct current through an electroresistant metal electrode to heat the electrode (much like an incandescent light bulb).[1] The heated electrode is applied to tissue to cause thermal necrosis and hemocoagulation to effect hemostasis. This technique does not pass electrical current through the patient and does not cause significant electromagnetic interference with implanted electrical devices, such as defibrillators and pacemakers. Most often the electrocautery units are small, battery powered, and appropriate for superficial or small mucosal or dermal bleeders.[66] Various power setting and tip sizes control the temperature of the tip. This and contact time determine lateral extent of tissue thermal necrosis.

Electrosurgery Unlike electrocautery, where a heated electrode is applied to tissue, electrosurgery actually passes electrons and hence electrical current through tissue. This application of electromotive energy caused local tissue heating and thermonecrosis. A high-frequency electrical generator using alternating current is used to increase standard wall outlet frequencies (approximately 60 Hz) to the 0.5-MHz to 3-MHz range. Electrical currents can be applied by monopolar or bipolar units.[67] In a monopolar unit, the current is passed from an electrode point, through the patient to a grounding pad. The electron density is much greater at the small electrode as opposed to the large grounding pad, so much more energy per unit area is delivered at the electrode. Monopolar units can be used in cutting mode (low-voltage uninterrupted alternating current [AC] causing cell explosion and limiting lateral thermal injury) or coagulation mode (interrupted AC at a higher voltage, causing greater lateral thermocoagulation and better hemostasis). Bipolar units use current passed between the 2 electrodes and the tissue between them and by their nature are more commonly used for hemostasis rather than surgical incisions. Additionally, monopolar units can be used to fulgurate tissue (where the electrode is held away from the tissue, causing electrical arcing between the electrode and tissue, leaving a char layer that is used for hemostasis over a broader area).[68]

Application of electrical current causes a plume that may spread infectious viral or prion particles, so that high-volume suction and protection of skin and mucosal surfaces are mandatory when using this modality. In addition, when in proximity to combustible material, electrical currents can generate a surgical site fire. As discussed previously, bipolar electrocautery may be a more appropriate hemostatic measure in a patient with an implanted electrical device because the electrical field is small and the current is not passed through the patient. If a monopolar device is necessary, placement of the grounding pad should be planned so that the current pathway is a far away from the implanted device as possible.[69]

Lasers

Laser is an acronym for light amplification by stimulated emission of radiation. Application of energy (often electrical current) to a medium causes the medium to emit monochromatic (1 wavelength) photons. A resonant chamber with reflective and partially transmissible mirrors produces a monochromatic beam that is coherent (all waves in phase) and collimated. Laser light wavelengths are selected to affect certain chromophores (portions of molecules that absorb the light energy).[70] Carbon-dioxide lasers use water as a chromophore and cause cellular disruption by intracellular vaporization. Depending on the confluence

Table 1
Commonly available topical hemostatic agents

Classification	Product	Trade Name	Manufacturer	Approximate Price
Scaffold/matrix	Gelatin matrix	Gelfoam Dental Sponge 2 × 2 cm	Pfizer	$205.90 (package of 6)
		Surgifoam Oral 1 × 1 cm	Ethicon	$180 (package of 24)
	Microfibrillar collagen	Avetine Flour	Bard Davol	$225 (1-g package)
		CollaPlug	Zimmer	$150 (package of 10)
	Oxidize cellulose	Surgicel 1.3 × 5 cm	Ethicon	$496 (package of 12)
	Mucopolysaccharide spheres	Arista-AH	Bard Davol	$2350 (3-g syringe, package of 5)
Biological	Thrombin, bovine	Thrombin-JMI (Pfizer, New York, NY)	Pfizer	$120 (5000-U vial)
	Thrombin, human pooled	Evithrom (Pfizer, New York)	Ethicon	$100 (5000-U vial)
	Thrombin, human recombinant	Recothrom (Bristol Meyers Squibb, New York)	Bristol Meyers Squibb	$61 (5000-U vial)
Antifibrinolytics	EACA	Amicar (Xanodyne, Newport, KY) 25% rinse	Xanodyne	$40/g (tablets) (pharmacy compounded)
	TA	Cyklokapron (Pfizer, New York, NY) 5% rinse	Pfizer	$50/g (intravenous injectable)
Natural propcoagulants	Chitosan	HemeCon T(Tricol Biomedical, Portland, OR)	Medical Technologies	$20 (7.6 cm × 3.6 m package)
	Zeolite	QuickClot (Z-Medica LLC, Wallingford, CT) ACS Sponge	Z -Medica	$30 (1/package)
	Alginate	Sorbsan (Mylan Bertek, Canonsburg, PA)	Bertek	$53 (12 in rope, package of 5)
	Hydrophilic polymers/K salts	BioSeal CVC Powder	BioLife	$32.00 (1 application package)
	Mineral salts	Aluminum chloride solution	Pharmacy compounded	—
		Zinc chloride solution	Pharmacy compounded	—
Tissue sealants	Thrombin + fibrinogen	Tisseel (Baxter, Deerfield, IL)	Baxter	$250.00 (2-mL kit)
	Bovine gelatin + thrombin	FloSeal (Baxter, Deerfield, IL)	Baxter	$190.00 (2-mL syringe)
Tissue adhesives	Cyanoacrylate	Histoacryl (B Braun USA, Bethlehem, PA)	Aesculap	$560 (package of 10)
		Dermabond (Ethicon US LLC, Somerville NJ)	Ethicon	$33 (0.7-mL syringe)
		Surgiseal (Adhezion Biomedical, Hudson, NC)	Achezion Biomedical	$200 (0.35-mL syringe; 12/ package)
	Polyethylene glycol hydrogel	CoSeal (Baxter, Deerfield, IL)	Baxter	$400 (2-mL syringe)
	Bovine albumin cross-linked	BioGlue (CryoLife, Kennesaw, GA)	CryoLife	$700 (5-mL delivery system)

(continued on next page)

Table 1 (continued)				
Classification	Product	Trade Name	Manufacturer	Approximate Price
Occlusives	Bone wax (Ethicon US LLC, Somerville, NJ)		Ethicon	$340 (2.5-g stick, 12/ box)
	Ostene (Baxter, Deerfield, IL)		Baxter	$980 (2.5-g stick, 12/ box)

(amount of joules per unit area) delivered and duration of incident laser energy, lateral tissue coagulation can yield hemostasis. Pulsing these lasers can limit lateral tissue thermal damage but also may limit hemorrhage control of larger vessels. Also, carbon-dioxide lasers cannot be used in fluid-filled spaces (such as joints) because the fluid itself, not the target tissue, absorbs the laser light energy. Unpulsed carbon-dioxide laser surgery, however, is generally considered an excellent tool for relatively bloodless incisions and control of bleeding from vessels less than 1 mm in diameter.[71] Care must be taken to provide eye protection for all operating room personnel as well as limit the presence of combustible materials in the field. Like electrical hemostatic techniques, protection for a potentially infective vaporized plume must be in place. Minimal use of open-airway supplemental oxygen or the use of laser-save endotracheal tubes is advocated when using carbon-dioxide lasers for surgery to minimize fire hazard.[72] Holmium/YAG lasers have been found useful in intra-articular arthroscopic surgery because the laser light can be transmitted through a fiberoptic cable and, when used in noncontact mode in a pulsed manner, the wavelength has sufficient tissue absorption to cause both ablation and hemostasis with much less water energy absorption than the carbon-dioxide laser, as long as continuous intra-articular irrigation can be maintained.[73]

SUMMARY

The choice of hemostatic modality depends on the amount of expected or actual bleeding encountered and any possible bleeding diathesis in the patient history. Most often, simple direct measures (topical or digital pressure to allow artery retraction, hemostat application, and vessel ligation) or a hypotensive technique can minimize surgical blood loss. Specific topical hemostatic agents and techniques may be useful adjuncts with many maxillofacial surgery applications. When considering their use, the increased cost of more recently developed modalities must be balanced against their often improved side-effect profile (**Table 1**). The ever-expanding armamentarium of topical hemostatic agents and techniques may prove useful, however, in both office-based and major operating room–based procedures.

REFERENCES

1. Moghandam H, Caminiti M. Life-threatening hemorrhage after extraction of third molars: case report and management protocol. J Can Dent Assoc 2002;68(11):670–4.
2. Schneider KM, Altay MA, Demko C, et al. Predictors of blood loss during orthognathic surgery: outcomes from a teaching institution. Oral Maxillofac Surg 2015;19(4):361–7.
3. Al-Sebaei ML. Predictors of intra-operative blood loss and blood transfusion in orthognathic surgery: A retrospective cohort study in 92 patients. Patient Saf Surg 2014;8(1):41.
4. Weber RS. A model for predicting transfusion requirement in head and neck surgery. Laryngoscope 1995;105(8 Pt 2 Suppl 73):1–17.
5. Leung L. Overview of hemostasis. Up To Date; 2015. Available at: http://www.uptodate.com/contents/overview-of-hemostasis?source=search_result&search=review+of+hemostasis&selectedTitle=3%7E150.
6. Hansson K, Stenflo J. Post-translational modification in proteins involved in blood coagulation. J Thromb Haemost 2005;3:2633.
7. Triplett D. Coagulation and bleeding disorders: review and update. Clin Chem 2000;46(8):1260–9.
8. Hong YM, Loughlin KR. The use of hemostatic agents and sealants in urology. J Urol 2006;176:2367.
9. Council on Pharmacy and Chemistry. Absorbable gelatin sponge: new and nonofficial remedies. J Am Med Assoc 1947;135:921.
10. Gelfoam [package insert]. Kalamazoo, Mich: Pharmacia; 1999.
11. Zucker WH, Mason RG. Ultrastructural aspects of interactions of platelets with microcrystalline collagen. Am J Pathol 1976;82:129–42.

12. Qerimi B, Baumann P, Hüsing J, et al. Collagen hemostat significantly reduces time to hemostasis compared with cellulose: COBBANA, a single-center, randomized trial. Am J Surg 2013;205:636.

13. Zimmer regenerative products catalog. 2015. Available at: http://www.dentalglam.ee/public/files/zimmer_Regenerative_Products.pdf. Accessed 2015.

14. Sharma JB, Malhorta M. Topical oxidized cellulose for tubal hemorrhage hemostasis during laparoscopic sterilization. Int J Gynaecol Obstet 2003; 82:221.

15. Spangler D, Rothenburger S, Nguyen K, et al. In vitro antimicrobial activity of oxidized regenerated cellulose against antibiotic-resistant microorganisms. Surg Infect (Larchmt) 2003;4(3):255–62.

16. Ibrahim MF, Aps C, Young CP. A foreign body reaction to Surgicel mimicking an abscess following cardiac surgery. Eur J Cardiothorac Surg 2002;22: 489–90.

17. Bard Davol product brochure. Available at: http://www.davol.com/Slatwall/custom/assets/files/product brochure/DAV-2127-Arista%20Brochure_app.pdf. Accessed 2016.

18. Antisdell JL, Janney CG, Long JP, et al. Hemostatic agent microporous polysaccharide hemospheres (MPH) does not affect healing of intact sinus mucosa. Laryngoscope 2008;118(7):1265–9.

19. Galarza M, Porcar OP, Gazzeri R, et al. Microporous polysaccharide hemospheres (MPH) for cerebral hemostasis: a preliminary report. World Neurosurg 2011;75(3–4):491–4.

20. Lewis KM, Atlee H, Mannone A, et al. Efficacy of hemostatic matrix and microporous polysaccharide hemospheres. J Surg Res 2015;193(2):1016.

21. Lawson JH, Lynn KA, Vanmatre RM, et al. Antihuman factor V antibodies after use of relatively pure bovine thrombin. Ann Thorac Surg 2005;79:1037–8.

22. Chapman WC, Singla N, Genyk Y, et al. A phase 3, randomized, doubleblind comparative study of the efficacy and safety of topical recombinant human thrombin and bovine thrombin in surgical hemostasis. J Am Coll Surg 2007;205:256–65.

23. Aronson J. Meyler's side effects of drugs. 16th edition. Amsterdam: Elsevier; 2016. p. 213–5.

24. Dubber AH, McNicol GP, Douglas AS, et al. Some properties of the antifibrinolytically active isomer of aminomethylcyclohexane carboxylic acid. Lancet 1964;2:1317.

25. Sindet-Pedersen S, Stjenberg S. Effect of local antifibrinolytic treatment with tranexamic acid in hemophiliacs undergoing oral surgery. J Oral Maxillofac Surg 1986;44:703–7.

26. Carter G, Goss A. Tranexamic acid mouthwash-A prospective randomized study of a 2-day regimen vs 5-day regimen to prevent postoperative bleeding in anticoagulated patients requiring dental extractions. Int J Oral Maxillofac Surg 2003;32:504–7.

27. van Diermen D, van der Waal I, Hoogstraten J. Management recommendations for invasive dental treatment in patient using oral antithrombotic medication, including novel oral anticoagulants. Oral Surg Oral Med Oral Pathol Oral Radiol 2013;116:709–16.

28. Shenoy A, Ramesh KV, Chowta MN, et al. Effects of botropase on clotting factors in healthy human volunteers. Perspect Clin Res 2014;5(2):71–4.

29. Eftekharian H, Vahedi R, Karagah T, et al. Effect of tranexamic acid irrigation on perioperative blood loss during orthognathic surgery: a double-blind, randomized controlled clinical trial. J Oral Maxillofac Surg 2015;73(1):129–33.

30. Joshi S, Gadre KS, Halli R, et al. Topical use of hemocoagulase (Reptilase): a simple and effective way of managing post-extraction bleeding. Ann Maxillofac Surg 2014;4(1):119.

31. Majumder K. Efficacy of haemocoagulase as a topical haemostatic agent after minor oral surgical procedures: a prospective study. Int J Clin Med 2014;5:875–83.

32. Chan MW, Schwaitzberg SD, Demcheva M, et al. Comparison of poly-N-acetyl glucosamine with absorbable collagen (Actifoam) and fibrin sealant (BioHeal)for achieving hemostasis in a swine model of splenic temorrhage. J Trauma 2000;48: 454–7.

33. Jayakumar R, Prabaharan M, Sudheesh Kumar PT, et al. Biomaterials based on chitin and chitosan in wound dressing applications. Biotechnol Adv 2011;29(3):332–7.

34. Griffin J. Role of surface in surface-dependant activation of Hageman factor (blood coagulation factor XII). Proc Natl Acad Sci U S A 1978;75:1998–2002.

35. Auchneck H, Sileshi B, Jamiolkowski RM, et al. A comprehensive review of topical hemostatic agents: Efficacy and recommendations for use. Ann Surg 2010;251(2):217–28.

36. Segal H, Hunt B, Gilding K. The effects of alginate and non-alginate wound dressings on blood coagulation and platelet activation. J Biomater Appl 1998; 12(3):249–57.

37. Heenan A. Alginate dressings. Worldwide Wounds. Available at: http://www.worldwidewounds.com/1998/june/Alginates-FAQ/alginates-questions.html. Accessed 1998.

38. Kumar KS, Reddy GV, Naidu G, et al. Role of povidone iodine in periapical surgeries: Hemostyptic and anti-inflammatory? Ann Maxillofac Surg 2011; 1(2):107–11.

39. WoundSeal fact sheet. Sarasota (FL): Biolife; 2012. Available at: http://woundseal.com/wp/faqs.

40. Ho J, Hruza G. Hydrophilic polymers with potassium salt and microporous polysaccharides for use as hemostatic agents. Dermatol Surg 2007;33:1430–3.

41. Palm M, Altman J. Topical hemostatic agents: a review. Dermatol Surg 2008;34(4):431–45.

42. Larson P. Topical hemostatic agents for dermatologic surgery. J Dermatol Surg Oncol 1988;14:623–32.

43. Epstein E, Mailbach H. Monsel's solution: history, chemistry, and efficacy. Arch Dermatol 1964;90:226–8.

44. Mohs F. Chemosurgery: a method for the microscopically controlled excision of cancer of the skin and lips. Geriatrics 1959;14:77–88.

45. Brown O, Goldstein G, Rirkby C. Auto-Mohs. Dermatol Surg 2001;27:275–8.

46. Sawchuck W, Friedman KJ, Manning T, et al. Delayed healing in full-thickness wounds treated with aluminum chloride solution. A histologic study with evaporimetry correlation. J Am Acad Dermatol 1985;15:982–99.

47. Silvergleid A. Fibrin sealant. Up To Date; 2015. Available at: http://www.uptodate.com/contents/fibrin-sealant?source=see_link.

48. Soffer E, Ouhayoun JP, Anagnostou F. Fibrin sealants and platelet preparations in bone and periodontal healing. Oral Surg Oral Med Oral Pathol Oral Radiol Endod 2003;95:521.

49. Albanese A, Licata ME, Polizzi B, et al. Platelet rich plasma (PRP) in dental and oral surgery: from the wound healing to bone regeneration. Immun Ageing 2013;10:23.

50. Zollino I, Candotto V, Silvestre FX, et al. Efficacy of platelet rich plasma in oral surgery and medicine: an overview. Ann Oral Maxillofac Surg 2014;2(1):5.

51. Ramos-Torrecillas J, De Luna-Bertos E, García-Martínez O, et al. Clilnical utility of growth factors and platelet-rich plasma in tissue regeneration: a review. Wounds 2014;26(7):207–13.

52. Singer AJ, Quinn JV, Hollander JE. The cyanoacrylate topical skin adhesives. Am J Emerg Med 2000;18:511.

53. Toriumi D, Bagal A. Cyanoacrylate tissue adhesives for skin closure in the outpatient setting. Otolaryngol Clin North Am 2002;35:103.

54. Hagberg R, Safi HJ, Sabik J, et al. Improved intraoperative management of anastamotic bleeding during aortic reconstruction: results of a randomized controlled trial. Am Surg 2004;70:307–11.

55. Coagrove G, Delashaw JB, Grotenhuis JA, et al. Safety and efficacy of a novel polyethylene glycol hydrogel sealant for watertight dural repair. J Neurosurg 2007;106:52–8.

56. Sidle DM, Loos B, Ramierz A, et al. Use opf BioGlue surgical adhesive for brow fixation in endoscopic browplasty. Arch Facial Plast Surg 2005;7:393–7.

57. Qayum A, Koka A. Foreign body reaction to bone wax: an unusual casue of persistent serous discharge from iliac crest graft donor site and the possible means to avoid such complication. A case report. Cases J 2009;2:9097.

58. Gibbs L, Kakis A, Weinstein P, et al. Bone wax as a risk factor for surgical site infection following neurospinal surgery. Infect Control Hosp Epidemiol 2004;25:346.

59. Wang M, Armstrong JK, Fisher TC, et al. A new, pluronic-based bone hemostatic agent that does not impair osteogenesis. Neurosurgery 2001;49:962–7.

60. Wellisz T, Armstrong J, Cambridge J, et al. Ostene, a new water soluble bone hemostasis agent. J Craniofac Surg 2006;17(3):420–5.

61. Katzung B, Masters S, Trevor A. Basic and clinical pharmacology. New York: McGraw-Hill; 2009.

62. Firoz B, Davis N, Goldberg LH. Local anesthesia using buffered 0.5% lidocaine with 1:200,000 epinephrine for tumors of the digits treated with Mohs micrographic surgery. J Am Acad Dermatol 2009;61(4):639–43.

63. Klein JA. The tumescent technique for liposuction surgery. Am J Cosmet Surg 1987;4:263.

64. Potter J, Finn R, Cillo J. Modified tumescent technique for outpatient facial laser resurfacing. J Oral Maxillofac Surg 2004;62:829–33.

65. Pollock SV. Electrosurgery. Bolognia JL, Jorizzo JL, Rapini RP, editors. Dermatology. 2nd edition. St Louis (MO): Mosby Elsevier; 2009. p. 2303–12. Ch140.

66. Lane JE, O'brien EM, Kent DE. Optimization of thermocautery in excisional dermatologic surgery. Dermatol Surg 2006;32(5):669–75.

67. Massarweh N, Cosgriff N, Slakey D. Electrosurgery: history, principles, and current and future uses. J Am Coll Surg 2006;202(3):520.

68. Einarsson J, Gould J. Overview of electrosurgery. Up To Date; 2016. Available at: http://www.uptodate.com/contents/overview-of-electrosurgery#references.

69. Chauvin M, Crenner F, Brechenmacher C. Interactoin between permanent cardiac pacing and electrocautery: the significance of electrode position. Pacing Clin Electrophysiol 1992;15:2028–35.

70. Nelson J, Berns M. Basic laser physics and tissue interactions. Contemp Dermatol 1988;2:1–20.

71. Rao G, Tripthi P, Srinivassen K. Hemostatic effect of the OW2 laser over escision of an intraoral hemangioma. Int J Laser Dent 2012;2(3):74–7.

72. OSHA Guidelines for laser safety and hazard assessment. OSHA; 1991. Available at: https://www.osha.gov/pls/oshaweb/owadisp.show_document?p_id=1705&p_table=DIRECTIVES.

73. Kaneyama K, Segami N, Sato J, et al. Outcomes of 152 temporomandibular joints following arthroscopic anterolateral capsular release by holmium:YAG laser or electrocautery. Oral Surg Oral Med Oral Pathol Oral Radiol Endod 2004;97:546–51.

Interventional Radiology and Bleeding Disorders
What the Oral and Maxillofacial Surgeon Needs to Know

Laura Gart, DMD[a], Antoine M. Ferneini, MD[b,c],*

KEYWORDS

- Embolization • Angiography • Bleeding • AV malformation • Epistaxis • Endovascular techniques
- Orthognathic surgery • TMJ ankylosis

KEY POINTS

- Endovascular techniques are essential for controlling acute head and neck bleeding that cannot be controlled by local or systemic measures.
- Angiography is the gold standard for the diagnosis and localization of acute head and neck bleeding.
- The oral and maxillofacial surgeon should refer a patient for an embolization procedure if local measures fail to achieve hemostasis.

INTRODUCTION

Hemostasis in the normal patient population involves the interaction among four different biologic systems: (1) the blood vessel wall, (2) the blood platelets, (3) the coagulation cascade, and (4) the fibrinolytic system. Hemostasis occurs through two independent processes: the coagulation cascade and the platelet activation pathway.[1] Most perioperative bleeding in the maxillofacial region is usually controlled with local measures. Suggested management to control hemorrhage in the head and neck area includes unipolar and bipolar electrocautery, laser ablation, local anesthetics with vasoconstrictors, and direct pressure. However, when bleeding cannot be controlled with local measures, endovascular techniques are indicated to achieve adequate hemostasis.

Uncontrollable epistaxis is another bleeding state that may be encountered in patients. Most cases (70%) are idiopathic, but epistaxis can occur secondary to trauma; tumor; radiotherapy; coagulopathy; or vascular malformations or diseases, such as Osler-Weber-Rendu disease.

Another potential source of bleeding in surgical patients includes arteriovenous malformations (AVMs). Endovascular technology is actually used before surgical resection. More recently, this technology is used to provide complete and persistent occlusion of mandibular AVMs.[2] AVMs are classified based on their blood flow characteristics. AVMs contain enlarged torturous arteries and veins with collateralization from contralateral vessels. The pressure differential compared with the surrounding tissues created by the low-pressure vascular channel creates an environment where rapid shunting and recruitment of peripheral vessels can occur.[3] They are described as high-flow or low-flow. Lesions containing arteries are typically high-flow. Lesions consisting of capillary, venous, lymphatic, and venous-lymphatic

[a] Division of Oral and Maxillofacial Surgery, Yale-New Haven Hospital, 333 Cedar St, New Haven, CT 06510, USA; [b] Private Practice, Connecticut Vascular Center, PC, 280 State St, North Haven, CT 06473, USA; [c] Division of Vascular Surgery, Yale-New Haven Hospital/St. Raphael Campus, 1450 Chapel St, New Haven, CT, 06511, USA
* Corresponding author. Private Practice, Connecticut Vascular Center, PC, 280 State St, North Haven, CT 06473, USA
E-mail address: aferneini@ctvascularcenter.com

Oral Maxillofacial Surg Clin N Am 28 (2016) 533–542
http://dx.doi.org/10.1016/j.coms.2016.06.012
1042-3699/16/© 2016 Elsevier Inc. All rights reserved.

malformations are generally low-flow.[3,4] High-flow lesions have the greatest potential for morbidity and mortality, thus making them more difficult to treat. Severe bleeding or exsanguination may often result with these high-flow lesions.

A considerable risk for hemorrhage exists in temporomandibular joint (TMJ) ankylosis surgery. During TMJ ankylosis surgery, many vessels that lie near the medial aspect of the condylar neck are traumatized. Vessels in the pterygoid fossa are a potential bleeding source during surgery. Branches of the maxillary artery and the pterygoid venous plexus can often be sources of hemorrhage. When compression alone fails to stop the bleeding, interventional radiology is a useful tool to control bleeding that the oral and maxillofacial surgeon may encounter in the operating room.[5] Complications associated with TMJ ankylosis surgery include damage to vascular structures. Methods used to achieve hemostasis include electrocautery, laser ablation, local anesthetics with vasoconstrictors, direct pressure, embolization, and ligation.[6] The middle meningeal and maxillary arteries are injured with a minimum amount of trauma.[7] To control the bleeding, pressure should be first applied at the surgical site with packing and manipulation of the systemic blood pressure. If bleeding does not stop with pressure, electrocautery is used. If cautery is not enough, coagulation products, such as topical thrombin or oxidized cellulose, are used. If hemorrhage has not stopped with these measures, the external carotid artery (ECA) is ligated above the level of the facial artery, or fluoroscopic embolization is considered.[7] Additionally, if intraoperative bleeding is a concern, preoperative angiography and embolization are performed to localize and embolize the vessels.[8]

Endovascular technology is also used in orthognathic surgery intraoperatively to control hemorrhage and postoperative. Excessive bleeding and injury to the internal maxillary artery, although uncommon, can occur during orthognathic surgery. The inferior alveolar branch of the internal maxillary artery is vulnerable to injury when osteotomies are made. Intraoperatively, one of the first measures to control intraoperative hemorrhage includes conservative measures, such as manipulating the systemic blood pressure and pressure. Packing should be used as the first attempt to tamponade the hemorrhage. In the presence of hypovolemic shock and if conservative measures have failed, intraoperative hemorrhage is controlled via transcatheter arterial embolization or ligation.[9] Additionally, a complication of orthognathic surgery includes the formation of a pseudoaneurysm, usually 1 to 8 weeks postoperatively.[10,11] A pseudoaneurysm is treated with embolization and microcoils. Pseudoaneurysm of the ECA or one of its branches is rare. In a series of more than 8000 aneurysms, 21 pseudoaneurysms of the ECA were described, 19 of which occurred after surgery in the region of the carotid artery.[12] The rarity of an ECA pseudoaneurysm is caused by the small size of the ECA branches, which makes cross-cutting more likely than a partial laceration. Pseudoaneurysms after orthognathic surgery are also rare. The literature includes about 18 case reports of pseudoaneurysms after orthognathic surgery.[11] Depending on the side of bleeding, a selective angiogram of the ECA (of the affected side) is usually performed. Embolization can then be achieved. The goal of embolization is to deposit an embolic material within the aneurysmatic network and not to compromise the vascular supply near the injury.[13] Endovascular treatment has been used to treat pseudoaneurysms of the descending palatine artery and internal maxillary artery.[11,14] Endovascular methods to control hemorrhage are discussed in this article.

ENDOVASCULAR TECHNIQUES

Endovascular techniques have played a major role in the management of head and neck bleeding and lesions since selective embolization of the ECA was described by Djindjian and colleagues[15] in 1972. Embolotherapy or embolization has rapidly developed in recent years and is now standard of care in most hospital centers. It is defined as the percutaneous application of one or more of a variety of agents or materials to accomplish vascular occlusion and bleeding control. Embolotherapy has evolved over the past 10 years and includes a wide variety of clinical applications, including the following:

1. Vascular malformations: occlusion of congenital or acquired aneurysms (cerebral, visceral, or extremities), vascular malformations, and pseudoaneurysms.
2. Trauma: for control of acute hemorrhage or uncontrollable bleeding.
3. Uterine artery embolization: either to reduce intraoperative blood loss or devascularization of benign uterine leiomyomas.
4. Nontraumatic hemorrhage: caused by either acute or recurrent hemorrhage. This includes hemoptysis, gastrointestinal bleeding, postpartum hemorrhage, and hemorrhagic neoplasms.
5. Oncologic embolization: either palliative or curative. Embolization is performed to prevent or treat hemorrhage, relieve symptoms, reduce intraoperative blood loss, improve quality of life, and improve survival. Examples include renal cell carcinoma, primary and secondary bone malignancies, and various hepatic malignancies.

6. Tissue ablation: ablation of benign neoplastic and nonneoplastic tissue. This includes hypersplenism, varicocele, pelvic congestion syndrome, priapism, and abdominal pregnancy.
7. Flow redistribution: to protect normal tissue. For example, gastroduodenal artery and right gastric artery embolization in hepatic artery chemoembolization and radioembolization.
8. Regional therapy delivery: as a vehicle for delivery of drugs and other agents. This includes chemotherapy, β-emiting spheres, and oncolytic viruses.
9. Endoleak management: this includes direct sac puncture or collateral vessel embolization.

Endovascular techniques are the standard of care to diagnose and treat maxillofacial bleeding. It plays a major role in acute bleeding and AVMs. Simple curettage of AVMs alone carries high risks of morbidity, mortality, and recurrence (**Fig. 1**). Ligation (eg, ECA) or endovascular occlusion are methods that should not be used because they do not control the bleeding due to the ability of the lesion to rapidly recruit collateral vessels.

In addition, intra-arterial embolization alone is often ineffective because the arterial pedicles occlude before complete filling of the venous pouch, leading to a high recurrence rate. Thus, new techniques in interventional radiology have been developed to replace the often ineffective surgical and endovascular occlusion methods.

New techniques in interventional radiology include the percutaneous treatment method. This method with possible use of embolization has proven to reduce the need for surgical intervention.[3,16,17] Highly selective embolization has been used to decrease blood flow to AVMs, but there is still a high risk for bleeding. The reason for this is that collateral vessels are recruited from the contralateral circulation or from branches of the internal carotid artery (ICA).[3]

Percutaneous or transosseous direct puncture of the lesion directly accesses the lesion's nidus to limit blood flow and limit the morbidity and mortality that are inherent to these lesions. The lesion's central varix is completely irradiated and the lesion is hemostatic through the use of thrombogenic or sclerosing agents.[3] The surrounding lesion is

A

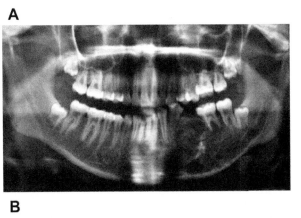

B

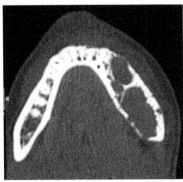 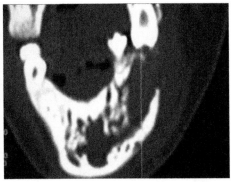

Fig. 1. (*A*) Preoperative orthopantogram showing moth-eaten irregular radiolucency in left mandibular parasymphysis body region with enlarged and torturous mandibular canal; adjacent teeth are displaced. (*B*) Axial computed tomography and coronal computed tomography section demonstrating widespread destruction and thinning of cortical plates. (*From* Singh V, Bhardwaj PK. Arteriovenous malformation of mandible: extracorporeal curettage with immediate replantation technique. Natl J Maxillofac Surg 2010;1(1):46; with permission.)

resected if bleeding persists, with less blood loss and morbidity and mortality than the traditional methods of embolization and resection. Surgery is performed within 24 to 48 hours of the embolization.

ANGIOGRAPHY

Angiography is the gold standard for the diagnosis and localization of acute bleeding. Angiography is considered a noninvasive standard procedure for a comprehensive imaging of the anatomy of the vasculature of the head and neck (**Figs. 2** and **3**). It is the next step once medical management has failed to control an active bleed. It allows for the use of embolization and vasopressin infusion when other management options have failed. Angiography allows the medical team to diagnose and formulate a treatment plan to achieve hemostasis.

Both the site and the source of bleeding are identified through this imaging modality. Angiography has proven to be an accurate diagnostic tool. This diagnostic imaging is used to accurately assess the flow characteristics and feeding vessel anatomy. For example, studies have shown that angiography can detect flow rates of 0.3 mL/min and has a sensitivity of 50% to 86% and specificity of 92% to 95% for identifying lesions associated with gastrointestinal bleeds.[18] It is difficult to detect venous bleeding with angiography.[19] Angiography is used for surgical planning and confirmation following surgery that the AVM was completely removed or that hemostasis is achieved (**Fig. 4**).[20]

In some cases, it may be necessary to perform computed tomography angiography imaging study to further characterize a hemorrhagic lesion. Technetium 99m–labeled red blood cell or technetium 99m sulfur colloid scintigraphy is used in computed tomography angiography to detect and localize bleeding.[19] Red cell scintigraphy can allow for delayed scans up to 24 hours after the radioisotope is injected. Injection with radionuclides has a false localization rate of 22%.[19] Metallic artifacts may also interfere with the visualization of the contrast and can lead to false-positive results.[19]

EMBOLIZATION

Embolization procedures for bleeding disorders in the head and neck region are mostly performed for intractable epistaxis, intraoperative hemorrhage (during orthognathic surgery or TMJ ankylosis surgery), or in the presence of a hypervascular tumor either before surgical removal or as a palliative treatment.[21] Indications for endovascular embolization include occlusion of unresectable lesions, staged occlusion for eventual resection, and emergent preoperative hemostatic control. Embolization has proven to be quite successful. The cure rate achieved in most reported series is 80% or higher, particularly when the ipsilateral facial artery and contralateral sphenopalatine artery are simultaneously embolized.[22–26]

Embolization can be performed under local anesthesia. However, most cases are performed under conscious sedation. However, general anesthesia is usually used in embolization

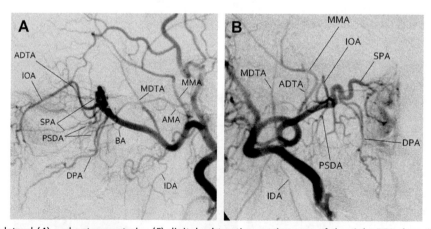

Fig. 2. Left lateral (*A*) and anteroposterior (*B*) digital subtraction angiograms of the right ECA show the first and second segments (*A*) and third segment (*B*) of the maxillary artery. ADTA, anterior deep temporal artery; AMA, accessory meningeal artery; BA, buccal artery; DPA, descending palatine artery; IDA, inferior dental artery; IOA, infraorbital artery; MDTA, middle deep temporal artery; MMA, middle meningeal artery; PSDA, posterior superior dental artery; SPA, sphenopalatine artery. (*From* Tanoue S, Kiyosue H, Mori H, et al. Maxillary artery: functional and imaging anatomy for safe and effective transcatheter treatment. Radiographics 2013;33(7):e212; with permission.)

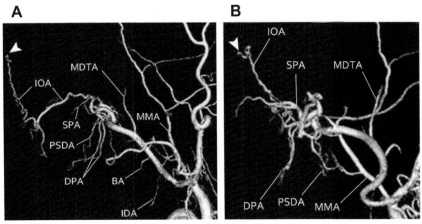

Fig. 3. Three-dimensional anatomy of the maxillary artery in a patient with an ethmoidal dural arteriovenous fistula. Left lateral (*A*) and anteroposterior (*B*) volume-rendered images from rotational angiographic data clearly depict the three-dimensional relationships of the maxillary artery and its branches. The arteriovenous fistula is fed by the left infraorbital artery (IOA) (*arrowhead*). BA, buccal artery; DPA, descending palatine artery; IDA, inferior dental artery; MDTA, middle deep temporal artery; MMA, middle meningeal artery; PSDA, posterior superior dental artery; SPA, sphenopalatine artery. (*From* Tanoue S, Kiyosue H, Mori H, et al. Maxillary artery: functional and imaging anatomy for safe and effective transcatheter treatment. Radiographics 2013;33(7):e231; with permission.)

procedures to control intraoperative bleeding. The embolization procedure requires four steps:

1. Percutaneous arterial access: either femoral or radial. The femoral artery has been the primary access. However, over the last 10 years, the radial artery has become popular. There are many advantages for a transradial access over a transfemoral access. These include the following:

    a. The radial artery is more superficial than the femoral one. Thus, there are no surrounding structures that are susceptible to injury. Additionally, an inadvertent injury to the artery itself is significantly less detrimental to the patient because of the dual blood supply to the hand.

    b. The radial artery is readily compressible, which decreases the incidence of postprocedural bleeding complications. Hemostasis is accomplished without the introduction of a foreign body, such as a vascular closure device.

    c. Postoperative care and patient comfort are usually easier with a transradial access. After a transradial access, patients can ambulate immediately, sit up, and usually have a quicker discharge.

2. Manipulation of catheters to selectively access the target vessel and use of catheters and microcatheters.

3. Handling and selection of various materials used for embolization.

4. Assessment of the angiographic or imaging modality to evaluate the therapeutic end point.

A wide variety of agents is available for the embolization of head and neck bleeding (**Box 1**). They are classified based on their physical state (liquid or solid), mechanism of action (mechanical vs chemical), and origin (autologous vs biosynthetic).[27] Several factors determine the correct agent for the given case. Particulate and

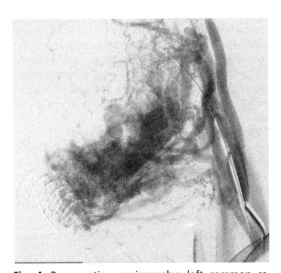

Fig. 4. Preoperative angiography: left common carotid angiogram, lateral projection, and arterial phase showing extensive mandibular AVM with arterial supply from multiple sources and drainage into the dilated inferior alveolar vein. (*From* Ferrés-Amat E, Prats-Armengol J, Maura-Solivellas I, et al. Gingival bleeding of a high-flow mandibular arteriovenous malformation in a child with 8-year follow-up. Case Rep Pediatr 2015;2015:745718; with permission.)

> **Box 1**
> **Available agents for the embolization of head and neck bleeding**
>
> *Particulate Agents: Absorbable*
> - Gelatin sponge particles
> - Gelatin sponge powder
> - Microfibrillar collagen
> - Autologous clot
>
> *Particulate Agents: Nonabsorbable*
> - Coils
> - Polyvinyl alcohol
> - Detachable balloons
> - Acrylic microspheres
>
> *Liquid Agents: Nonabsorbable*
> - Silicone
> - N-Butyl cyanoacrylate
> - Ethibloc
>
> *Liquid Agents: Cytotoxic*
> - Doxycycline
> - Sodium tetradecyl sulfate
> - Ethanol 95%
> - Chemotherapeutic agents

absorbable embolic agents are usually preferred to decrease the severity and longevity of potential ischemic events. Liquid and nonabsorbable agents are usually indicated for head and neck pathology where a more aggressive approach is indicated. The embolic materials most commonly used are particles, either of gelatin sponge or polyvinyl alcohol, and more recently trisacryl gelatin microspheres.[3,28]

The gelatin sponge is the most commonly used temporary embolic agent.[27] Gelatin sponge occludes the vessel for 3 to 6 weeks. The particle size can vary and vessels may be occluded causing ischemia. Gelatin sponge strips rolled into "torpedoes" are used to occlude larger vessels.

Microfibrillar collagen and oxidized cellulose are other temporary embolic agents that may be used. They are difficult to prepare, which makes them inferior to gelatin sponge. An autologous clot may also be considered an embolic agent in some cases, but because of its rapid lysis it has been shown to demonstrate little clinical success.[29] Recanalization of the vessel can occur in hours to days.

Polyvinyl alcohol particles are derived from inert plastic sponges. These particles are not resorbable. They adhere to the vessel wall and cause an inflammatory reaction and vessel fibrosis. The disadvantage of these particles is that they have a tendency to clump together and may occlude at a more proximal position than intended.[27] To avoid clumping of the particles, careful technique is needed, which includes proper suspension, dilution, slow infusion, and resuspension.

Another embolic agent that has been used is cyanoacrylate. The injection is continued into the bleeding area until no more angiographic shunt or bleeding occurs. Nonliquid embolization materials have also been used in embolization, which include gelatin sponge soaked in the thrombotic agent and a detachable balloon.[28] The use of coils is not recommended because proximal occlusion may not only induce the development of collateral circulation but also close the door to repeat access in case of recurrence.

The transcutaneous puncture embolization can also be performed with coils made of stainless steel or platinum that ideally completely fill the AVM. The coils come in straight, helical, spiral, and complex three-dimensional shapes and a range of diameters (submillimeters to several centimeters). The coils serve to decrease blood flow and increase turbulence in the AVMs.[3] They are less likely to migrate in lesions with high flow because of their great radial force.[27] The disadvantage with coils is the possibility for a partial obstruction because they rely on mechanical obstruction. Some coils may contain small fibers attached to the metal, which aids in the formation of a thrombus.[30] The coils rely on the patient's ability to form a clot and as a result their effectiveness may be unpredictable in coagulopathic states. This creates an environment where a clot can form.

Liquid embolic agents are more difficult to control. They function independently of the patient's coagulation system making them highly useful in patients with severe coagulopathies. Liquids can also reach beyond the catheter tip when bleeding sites may be difficult to reach. Examples of liquid embolic agents include ethanol, sodium tetradecyl sulfate, N-butyl cyanoacrylate, and ethylene vinyl copolymer.

For epistaxis, selective angiography of bilateral ICAs and ECAs is first performed with 4F or 5F catheters. ICA angiography is useful for evaluating any dangerous collateral vessels between the ECA and ICA and to delineate the predominant supply to the ophthalmic artery. Moreover, ICA injection also helps to delineate the ethmoidal artery supply to the nasal cavity. It is generally unsafe to embolize the anterior ethmoidal arteries with particulate agents because of the associated risk of blindness. The embolization is generally performed under systemic anticoagulation and with superselective catheterization of target vessels. We generally prefer microcatheters with larger bores (0.019–0.021 inches) and the use of 100 to 300 or 300 to 500 μm particles (Embospheres, Merit Medical Systems, Inc, South Jordan, UT) for embolization. The microcatheter is positioned just proximal to the branches supplying the nasal mucosa, and care is taken to avoid nontargeted vessel embolization. If smaller particles (100–300 μm) are chosen, they are typically used in small quantities because aggressive embolization with small particles is associated with a risk of necrosis of the embolized territory. Gelatin sponge pledgets may be placed in the vessel lumen after completing the embolization with particulate agents. Embolization is highly effective for treatment of intractable epistaxis with reported success rates ranging from 71% to 100%.[31–34] The most common cause of failure of this technique is bleeding from the anterior ethmoidal artery.[31–34]

The selection process for an ideal embolic agent includes consideration of vessel size, duration of occlusion desired, need for tissue viability (should the tissue supplied by the vessel remain viable after embolization), and patient's clinical condition.[35–37] Smaller embolic agents are more likely to occlude the primary and the collateral vessels. Duration of occlusion is important to consider when selecting an embolic agent. Embolic agents, such as autologous clots, may be present for a few hours, whereas nonresorbable liquid agents and metals may remain in place permanently.

POTENTIAL COMPLICATIONS OF THESE PROCEDURES

The most common complication encountered from embolization is headache or temporofacial pain, more common in cases where two or more arteries are embolized with gelatin sponge. Siniluoto and colleagues[17] reported that 96.8% of their patients experienced mild to moderate pain in the temporal area during the first 24 hours after embolization.[19,38]

Risks specific to transcutaneous puncture embolization include pulmonary embolism and cerebrovascular accident. It is possible for the coils to permeate through the venous outflow tract if the coils are too small.[39] Additional risks include necrosis or ischemia to surrounding vessels caused by decreased vascularity in the area and peripheral and central nervous system arterial spasm or vessel rupture. Other complications include groin hematoma, facial numbness, mucosal necrosis, and acute infection.

Soft tissue necrosis has also been reported as a complication, especially when more than one vessel is occluded (contralateral sphenopalatine artery or facial artery) or when liquid embolic agents are used. Small particles tend to produce a more distal occlusion and may also result in local ischemia and even nasal septal perforation.[40] At times, it is difficult to discern if the necrosis is secondary to the embolization procedure or to prolonged packing. Ischemic injury may not only affect the mucosa but also the cranial nerves, possibly resulting in temporary or permanent cranial nerve palsy.[41,42] Depending on the cranial nerve affected, the presenting symptoms are variable, including diplopia, dysphagia, and numbness. A cranial nerve examination is necessary preoperatively.

The most severe complications are those connected with the passage of embolic material into the intracranial arteries potentially leading to a stroke or blindness.[35,43] This may occur because of reflux from the ECA into the ICA or through the passage of embolic material through extracranial-intracranial anastomoses. At times, it may become necessary to perform selective embolization of branches originating from the ophthalmic artery. In this situation, the microcatheter should be advanced beyond the second portion of the ophthalmic artery to prevent embolic material from entering the central artery of the retina.[36]

In the presence of ipsilateral ICA stenosis or occlusion, the use of particles may be particularly dangerous because of the development of ECA to ICA anastomoses. In this situation, endovascular therapy may still be safely and effectively performed with coils in the pterygopalatine segment of the internal maxillary artery.[37]

Ligation of the ECA is no longer the treatment of choice for hemorrhage because continued bleeding can occur when collateral vessels are recruited from the contralateral ECA or the vertebral artery. Once the ECA is ligated, transarterial embolization is difficult. Embolization can take place if the distal part of the ligated ECA is surgically exposed and punctured. The challenge with this procedure is that the ECA becomes fibrotic at the ligation site and access to this vessel is difficult. There exists a high rate of complications associated with puncture of the ECA. Alternatively, embolization is performed using a transsuperficial temporal artery approach.[44] This method is also useful when other feeding vessels are too tortuous to be navigated with a catheter. Complications of this approach include damage to the superficial temporal nerve and vasospasm. Other methods also include transvenous embolization by direct

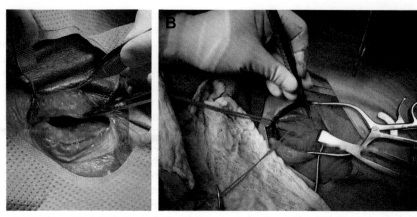

Fig. 5. (*A*) Neck dissection. (*B*) Bifurcation of the common carotid into the external and internal carotid arteries.

transosseous venous puncture or by transfemoral catheterization.

WHAT THE ORAL AND MAXILLOFACIAL SURGEON NEEDS TO KNOW

For most intraoperative and postoperative bleeding, local measures are usually adequate to achieve hemostasis. Angiography is now considered the gold standard to better localize the exact location of the bleeding. New techniques, such as direct transcutaneous puncture embolization, have been developed and can limit the morbidity and mortality associated with a coagulation defect. ECA ligation should be a last resort if embolization fails. The oral and maxillofacial surgeon should refer a patient for an embolization procedure if local measures fail to achieve hemostasis.

As a last resort, if hemostasis cannot be achieved, it may be necessary to unilaterally ligate the ECA (**Fig. 5**). Surgical ligation of the ECA is

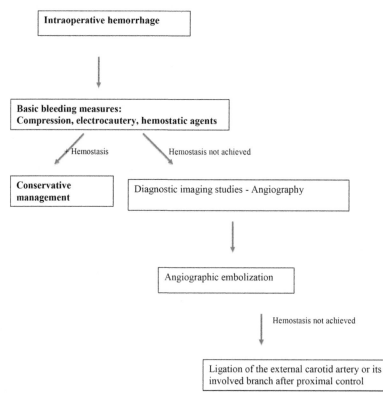

Fig. 6. Flow chart for acute hemorrhage.

performed safely without risk to cerebral perfusion.[44,45] Risks of ECA ligation include compromised arterial blood flow to the eye via the middle meningeal artery. Because of the extensive collateral circulation in the face, ligation at the origin of the ECA may not be effective, making ligation a less desirable approach to control hemostasis.[9]

In cases where the oral and maxillofacial surgeon needs to remove vascular lesions, such as angiofibromas and hypervascular metastases, microembolization may be indicated. Advantages include shorter operative times, reduced blood loss, and faster recovery.[46–48] Microembolization serves to selectively occlude the ECA feeders through intratumoral deposition of embolic material. Ideally, embolization is performed 24 to 72 hours before surgical thrombosis. This is an ideal time range to allow for thrombosis of the vessel and prevent recanalization of the occluded arteries or formation of collateral arterial channels. After a microcatheter is inserted into the artery that feeds the tumor, angiography of the ICA and ECA is performed. Caution must be exercised during the angiography because of the possibility for anastomoses between the ECA and ICA. Embolic material is then injected using fluoroscopic monitoring.[46] A major risk of embolization includes unintended ischemia in nonneoplastic tissue.[47]

SUMMARY

Endovascular techniques are essential for controlling acute head and neck bleeding that cannot be controlled by local or systemic measures (**Fig. 6**). Detailed knowledge of the head and neck vascular anatomy, advances in catheterization techniques, and the availability of new embolic materials have improved the safety, efficacy, and predictability of these techniques.

REFERENCES

1. Patton LL. Bleeding and clotting disorders. In: Greenberg MS, Glick M, Decker BC, editors. Burket's oral medicine: diagnosis and treatment. 10th edition. Hamilton (ON): BC Decker; 2003. p. 454–77.

2. Cohen JE, Gomori JM, Grigoriadis S, et al. Complete and persistent occlusion of arteriovenous malformations of the mandible after endovascular embolization. Neurol Res 2009;31(5):467–71.

3. Koebbe CJ, Horowitz M, Levy EI, et al. Endovascular particulate and alcohol embolization for near-fatal epistaxis from a skull base vascular malformation. Pediatr Neurosurg 2001;35(5):257–61.

4. Wehrli M, Lieberherr U, Valavanis A. Superselective embolization for intractable epistaxis: experiences with 19 patients. Clin Otolaryngol 1988;13: 415–20.

5. Kumar S, Bansal V, Agarwal R. An effective intraoperative method to control bleeding from vessels medial to the temporomandibular joint. J Maxillofac Oral Surg 2009;8(4):371.

6. Cillo JE Jr, Sinn D, Truelson JM. Management of middle meningeal and superficial temporal artery hemorrhage from total temporomandibular joint replacement surgery with a gelatin-based hemostatic agent. J Craniofac Surg 2005;16(2):309–12.

7. Dattilo DJ. Resection of the severely ankylosed temporomandibular joint. Atlas Oral Maxillofac Surg Clin North Am 2011;19(2):207–20.

8. Susarla SM, Peacock Z, Williams WB, et al. Role of computed tomographic angiography in treatment of patients with temporomandibular joint ankylosis. J Oral Maxillofac Surg 2014;72(2):267–76.

9. Khanna S, Dagum A. A critical review of the literature and an evidence-based approach for life-threatening hemorrhage in maxillofacial surgery. Ann Plast Surg 2012;69(4):474–8.

10. Manafi A, Ghenaati H, Dezham F, et al. Massive repeated nose bleeding after bimaxillary osteotomy. J Craniofac Surg 2007;18(6):1491–3.

11. Avelar RL, Goelzer JG, Becker OE, et al. Embolization of pseudoaneurysm of the internal maxillary artery after orthognathic surgery. J Craniofac Surg 2010;21(6):1764–8.

12. McCollum CH, Wheeler WG, Noon GP, et al. Aneurysm of the extracranial carotid artery. Twenty-one years' experience. Am J Surg 1979;137:196–200.

13. Zachariades N, Rallis G, Papademetriou G, et al. Embolization for the treatment of pseudoaneurysm and transection of facial vessels. Oral Surg Oral Med Oral Pathol Oral Radiol Endod 2001;92:491–4.

14. Fernandez-Prieto A, Garcia-Raya P, Burgueno M, et al. Endovascular treatment of a pseudoaneurysm of the descending palatine artery after orthognathic surgery: technical note. Int J Oral Maxillofac Surg 2005;34:321–3.

15. Djindjian R, Cophignon J, Théron J, et al. Embolization in vascular neuroradiology. Technique and indications apropos of 30 cases. Nouv Presse Med 1972;1(33):2153–8.

16. Tseng EY, Narducci CA, Willing SJ, et al. Angiographic embolization for epistaxis: a review of 114 cases. Laryngoscope 1998;108:615–9.

17. Siniluoto TMJ, Leinonen AS, Karttunen AI, et al. Embolization for the treatment of posterior epistaxis. Arch Otolaryngol Head Neck Surg 1993;119:837–41.

18. Chua AE, Ridley LJ. Diagnostic accuracy of CT angiography in acute gastrointestinal bleeding. J Med Imaging Radiat Oncol 2008;52(4):333–8.

19. Wu LM, Xu JR, Yin Y, et al. Usefulness of CT angiography in diagnosing acute gastrointestinal bleeding: a meta-analysis. World J Gastroenterol 2010;16(31): 3957–63.

20. Son YH, Baik SK, Kang MS, et al. Recurrent arteriovenous malformation on palate after embolization combined surgical resection: preoperative magnetic resonance features and intraoperative angiographic findings. J Korean Assoc Oral Maxillofac Surg 2015; 41(6):346–51.

21. Bilbao JI, Martínez-Cuesta A, Urtasun F, et al. Complications of embolization. Semin Intervent Radiol 2006;23:126–42.

22. Siu WWY, Weill A, Gariepy JL, et al. Arteriovenous malformation of the mandible: embolization and direct injection therapy. J Vasc Interv Radiol 2001; 12(9):1095–8.

23. Collette G, Valassina D, Bertossi D. Contemporary management of vascular malformations. J Oral Maxillofac Surg 2014;72:510.

24. Kohout MP, Hansen M, Pribaz JJ, et al. Arteriovenous malformations of the head and neck: natural history and management. Plast Reconstr Surg 1998;102(3):643–54.

25. Hyodoh H, Hori M, Akiba H, et al. Peripheral vascular malformations: imaging, treatment approaches, and therapeutic issues. Radiographics 2005;25:S159–71.

26. Resnick SA, Russell EJ, Hanson DH, et al. Embolization of a life-threatening mandibular vascular malformation by direct percutaneous transmandibular puncture. Head Neck 1992;14:372–9.

27. Medsinge A, Zajko A, Orons P, et al. A case-based approach to common embolization agents used in vascular interventional radiology. AJR Am J Roentgenol 2014;203(4):699–708.

28. Remonda L, Schroth G, Caversaccio M, et al. Endovascular treatment of acute and subacute hemorrhage in the head and neck. Arch Otolaryngol Head Neck Surg 2000;126(10):1255–62.

29. Lubarsky M, Ray CE, Funaki B. Embolization agents-which one should be used when? Part 1: large-vessel embolization. Semin Intervent Radiol 2009; 26(4):352–7.

30. Vaidya S, Tozer KR, Chen J. An overview of embolic agents. Semin Interv Radiol 2008;25(3):204–15.

31. Zheng JW, Mai HM, Zhang L, et al. Guideline for the treatment of head and neck venous malformations. Int J Clin Exp Med 2013;22:377.

32. Andersen PJ, Kjeldsen AD, Nepper-Rasmussen J. Selective embolization in the treatment of intractable epistaxis. Acta Otolaryngol 2005;125:293–7.

33. Layton KF, Kallmes DF, Gray LA, et al. Endovascular treatment of epistaxis in patients with hereditary hemorrhagic telangiectasia. AJNR Am J Neuroradiol 2007;28:885–8.

34. Strutz J, Schumacher M. Uncontrollable epistaxis, angiographic localization and embolization. Arch Otolaryngol Head Neck Surg 1990;116:697–9.

35. Mames RN, Snady-McCoy L, Guy J. Central retinal and posterior ciliary artery occlusion after particle embolization of the external carotid artery system. Ophthalmology 1991;98:527–31.

36. Sedat J, Dib M, Odin J, et al. Endovascular embolization of ophthalmic artery branches for control of refractory epistaxis. report of one case. J Radiol 2001;82:670–2.

37. Ernst RJ, Bulas RV, Gaskill-Shipley M, et al. Endovascular therapy of intractable epistaxis complicated by carotid artery occlusive disease. AJNR Am J Neuroradiol 1995;16:1463–8.

38. Oguni T, Korogi Y, Yasunaga T, et al. Superselective embolization for intractable idiopathic epistaxis. Br J Radiol 2000;73:1148–53.

39. Kademani D, Costello BJ, Ditty D, et al. An alternative approach to maxillofacial arteriovenous malformations with transosseous direct puncture embolization. Oral Surg Oral Med Oral Pathol Oral Radiol Endod 2004;97:701.

40. Coley S, Jackson JE. Pulmonary arteriovenous malformations. Clin Radiol 1998;53:396–404.

41. De Vries N, Versluis RJ, Valk J, et al. Facial nerve paralysis following embolization for severe epistaxis (case report and review of the literature). J Laryngol Otol 1986;100:207–10.

42. Low YM, Goh YH. Endovascular treatment of epistaxis in patients irradiated for nasopharyngeal carcinoma. Clin Otolaryngol 2003;28:244–7.

43. Elden L, Montanera W, Terbrugge K, et al. Angiographic embolization for the treatment of epistaxis: a review of 108 cases. Otolaryngol Head Neck Surg 1994;111:44–50.

44. Wang C, Yan Q, Xie X, Li J, et al. Embolization of a bleeding maxillary arteriovenous malformation via the superficial temporal artery after external carotid artery ligation. Korean J Radiol 2008;9(2): 182–5.

45. Abbas SM, Adams D, Vanniasingham P. What happens to the external carotid artery following carotid endarterectomy? BMC Surg 2008;8:20.

46. Gandhi D, Gemmete J, Ansari S, et al. Interventional neuroradiology of the head and neck. AJNR Am J Neuroradiol 2008;29:1806–15.

47. Macpherson P. The value of pre-operative embolization of meningiomas estimated subjectively and objectively. Neuroradiology 1991;33:334–7.

48. Dean BL, Flom RA, Wallace RC, et al. Efficacy of endovascular treatment of meningiomas: evaluation with matched samples. AJNR Am J Neuroradiol 1994;15:1675–80.

Blood Products
What Oral and Maxillofacial Surgeons Need to Know

Regina L. Landesberg, DMD, PhD[a],
Elie M. Ferneini, DMD, MD, MHS, MBA[b,c,d],*

KEYWORDS

- Fibrinogen concentrate • Transfusion complications • Anti-inhibitor coagulant complex
- Prothrombin complex concentrates • Cryoprecipitate • Fresh frozen plasma • Red blood cells
- Platelets

KEY POINTS

- Blood products are routinely used to manage various coagulation and hematological disorders.
- Oral and maxillofacial surgeons must have a basic knowledge and understanding of the various available products.
- A consultation with each patient's hematologist is always advised in order to decrease the risk of adverse events and improve the patient's safety.

INTRODUCTION

Blood products are used in the management of multiple coagulation disorders. However, there is a debate in the medical literature concerning the appropriate use of blood and blood products. Clinical trials investigating their use suggest that waiting to transfuse at lower hemoglobin levels is recommended.[1,2] Different products are available. A proper knowledge and understanding of the different blood products allows clinicians to optimize their patients' clinical outcomes.

RED BLOOD CELLS

Packed red blood cells (RBCs) are prepared from whole blood by removing 250 mL of plasma. One unit of packed RBCs should increase hemoglobin levels by 1 g/dL and hematocrit by 3%. In most areas, packed RBC units are filtered to reduce leukocytes before storage, which limits febrile nonhemolytic transfusion reactions, and are considered cytomegalovirus safe.[3]

RBC transfusions are used to treat hemorrhage as well as improve oxygen delivery to tissues. Transfusion of RBCs should be based on the patient's clinical condition.[4] Indications for RBC transfusion include:

- Restoration of oxygen-carrying capacity in case of acute hemorrhage: acute blood loss (>1500 mL or 30% of blood volume)
- Treatment of symptomatic anemia
- Prophylaxis in life-threatening anemia
- Exchange transfusion in different diseases, including:
  ○ Acute sickle cell crisis
  ○ Severe parasitic infection (malaria, babesiosis)
  ○ Severe methemoglobinemia
  ○ Severe hyperbilirubinemia of newborn

a Private Practice, Greater Waterbury OMS, 1389 West Main Street, Suite 320, Waterbury, CT 06708, USA;
b Private Practice, Greater Waterbury OMS, 435 Highland Avenue, Suite 100, Cheshire, CT 06410, USA;
c Beau Visage Med Spa, 435 Highland Avenue, Suite 100, Cheshire, CT 06410, USA; d Division of Oral and Maxillofacial Surgery, Department of Craniofacial Sciences, University of Connecticut, 263 Farmington Avenue, Farmington, CT 06030, USA
* Corresponding author. Beau Visage Med Spa, 435 Highland Avenue, Suite 100, Cheshire, CT 06410.
E-mail address: eferneini@yahoo.com

Oral Maxillofacial Surg Clin N Am 28 (2016) 543–552
http://dx.doi.org/10.1016/j.coms.2016.06.009
1042-3699/16/© 2016 Elsevier Inc. All rights reserved.

Recommended dosage and administration include:

- One unit of RBC increases the hemoglobin level of an average-sized adult by ~1 g/dL (or increases hematocrit ~3%)
- The ABO group of RBC products must be compatible with the ABO group of the recipient
- Ideally, the RBC product must be serologically compatible with the recipient
- Rate of transfusion
  - Transfuse slowly for the first 15 minutes
  - Complete transfusion within 4 hours (per US Food and Drug Administration [FDA])

The authors recommend transfusion when the hemoglobin level is less than 7 g/dL, and maintenance of a hemoglobin level between 7 and 9 g/dL.[1] Restrictive transfusion has been used since the late 1990s in most patients who do not have cardiac disease. An updated Cochrane Review supports the use of restrictive transfusion in patients without cardiac disease.[5] A randomized, multicenter, controlled clinical trial evaluated a restrictive transfusion trigger (hemoglobin level of 7–9 g/dL) versus a liberal transfusion trigger (hemoglobin level of 10–12 g/dL) in patients who are critically ill. Restrictive transfusion resulted in a 54% relative decrease in the number of units transfused and a reduction in the 30-day mortality. Another study compared restrictive with liberal transfusion and found similar results. The study showed that patients in the restrictive transfusion group received 44% fewer blood transfusions and there was no difference in rates of multiple organ dysfunction syndrome or death.[2] This type of transfusion is also helpful in stable pediatric patients in the intensive care unit.[2]

PLATELETS

In the United States, platelets are prepared by either apheresis or concentration of a whole-blood donation. Whole blood–derived platelet concentrates are prepared using the platelet-rich plasma method of double centrifugation with a resulting concentration of approximately 5.5×10^{10} platelets in 50 mL of plasma. The usual adult platelet transfusion pools 4 to 6 packs of whole-blood platelet concentrates. Apheresis units are obtained from a single platelet donor using an automated centrifugation unit that processes a high volume of blood. A typical apheresis unit should contain a minimum of 3×10^{11} platelets; the equivalent of 6 packs of pooled platelets. Apheresed platelet preparations are considered a leukoreduced blood product because they contain less than 5×10^6 white blood cells (WBCs) per unit.[6,7]

There are some minor advantages of apheresed platelets compared with whole blood–derived concentrates, most notably a longer survival time in the circulation,[8] which may be caused by gentler handling during preparation. Theoretically, there is less of a risk of viral transmission from apheresed platelets because apheresis units are derived from a single donor, whereas whole-blood platelet concentrates are pooled from 5 random donors. Improvements in screening blood donors have brought the risk of hepatitis B and C, and human immunodeficiency virus (HIV) to a minimum; however, bacterial contamination of platelet preparations has remained constant,[9] most likely because platelets, in contrast with other blood components, must be stored at room temperature because refrigerated platelets are cleared very rapidly from the circulation. However, room temperature storage increases the risk for bacterial growth. Limiting platelet holding time to only 5 days in most facilities is recommended.[10]

Although it was thought that apheresis platelets would elicit less exposure to alloantigens, and hence less alloimmunization, than pooled platelet preparations, clinical data did not support this hypothesis, possibly because platelet surface antigens are poor immunogens and the alloimmune response is caused by contaminating WBCs in the platelet preparation. Therefore, the use of leukoreduced platelets is likely to prevent this complication.[11]

Transfusion-related acute lung injury (TRALI) is associated with blood components that contain higher amounts of plasma, such as fresh frozen plasma (FFP) and platelets. The presence of donor anti–human leukocyte antigen (anti-HLA) (or less commonly antineutrophil) antibodies seems to precipitate this acute respiratory distress syndrome. Because a third of female blood donors have anti-HLA antibodies because of sensitization during pregnancy, it is tempting to limit platelet donations to only male patients in order to decrease the risk of TRALI from platelet transfusions. Although the production of FFP in the United States and several other countries is from male-only donors, assurance of adequate platelet supplies makes it necessary to continue to allow female donors.[9]

Platelet transfusions are currently used for prevention and treatment of bleeding in thrombocytopenic patients or in individuals with various platelet dysfunctions. A recent set of recommendations for platelet transfusions was established by the American Association of Blood Banks Task Force as well as the American Society of Anesthesiologists Task Force on Blood Component Therapy. However, clinical trials supporting these recommendations are lacking. The recommendations are shown in **Table 1**. Although the duration of

Table 1
Platelet transfusion recommendations

Indication	Platelets ($\times 10^9$/L)
Prevention of spontaneous bleeding in hospitalized patients	<10
Elective CVP placement	<20
Elective diagnostic lumbar puncture	<30
Major non-neurosurgical surgery	<50
Neurosurgical surgery	<100

Abbreviation: CVP, central venous port.

postsurgical platelet administration has not been well studied, it is generally accepted that monitoring and support for 7 days in moderate-risk to high-risk surgery is adequate.[12–15]

Inappropriately low platelet counts following multiple transfusions (platelet refractoriness) can be the result of immune and/or nonimmune causes. Fever, sepsis, medications, disseminated intravascular coagulation (DIC), splenomegaly, and bleeding are common causes of platelet refractoriness. Although antibodies to platelet HLA I antigens are the most common cause of immune-mediated platelet refractoriness, antibodies to platelet ABO and other platelet surface antigens have also been documented. Patients with 1-hour posttransfusional platelet counts that fail to achieve a corrected count increment of at least 5×10^9/L are candidates for either HLA-matched or crossmatched platelet transfusions.[9] However, a recent study that compared random donor HLA-matched and crossmatched platelet transfusions showed that neither of these therapies is as effective as was previously thought.[16]

PLASMA

Plasma is acellular and composed primarily of water (90%) and proteins (7%). The remaining 2% to 3% is made up of nutrients, crystalloids, hormones, and vitamins. The protein component contains the clotting factors von Willebrand factor (vWF); factor VIII (mostly bound to vWF); factor XIII; fibrinogen; and the vitamin K–dependent factors II, VII, IX, and X. Indications for the use of plasma product transfusions include conditions in which multiple coagulation defects exist, such as liver disease, massive transfusion, DIC, rapid reversal of warfarin, and replacement therapy for an inherited factor deficiency for which no factor concentrate exists or is available (factor II, V, X deficiencies). In addition, plasma products are used as a replacement fluid during plasma exchange

most commonly in the treatment of thrombotic thrombocytic purpura.[17]

At present, no evidence-based guidelines exist for the use of plasma administration in the conditions listed earlier; however, recent data from US military and civilian trauma centers have shown an increase in survival when trauma victims are resuscitated with a balanced ratio of RBCs/plasma/platelets.[18–20] In warfarin-anticoagulated patients who are actively bleeding or require emergency surgery, reversal with vitamin K (12–18 hours) is not an appropriate option. Because European prothrombin complex concentrate (PCC) preparations have higher concentrations of factor VII than in the United States, they can be used as the sole agents in rapid warfarin reversal. However, in the United States it is necessary to add plasma in addition to PCC for adequate therapy. Activated factor VII (factor VIIa) may also be useful for rapid warfarin reversal in patients with head injuries. International Normalized Ratio (INR) levels should be monitored closely in these patients and all of these therapies may carry an increased risk of thromboembolic events.[17]

FRESH FROZEN PLASMA, PLASMA FROZEN WITHIN 24 HOURS, THAWED PLASMA

FFP is prepared from freshly derived whole blood and must be frozen within 8 hours of collection. The resultant product is then stored at −18°C for up to 12 months and thawed over 20 to 30 minutes as needed. Plasma frozen within 24 hours of collection (PF24) is the most common plasma preparation used in the United States. The delay in freezing from 8 to 24 hours was recently evaluated and the data showed changes in activity levels, most notably of factor VII (−16%) and factor VIII (−15%). In contrast, vWF activity increased 34% and fibrinogen activity increased as well. However, all of the factors in thawed PF24 had activity levels greater than the minimum required for surgical hemostasis, supporting the use of either preparation when indicated. Thawed preparations of FFP and PF24 maintain factor levels that are considered safe for surgical hemostasis for up to 5 days when stored at 1 to 6°C.[17,21]

CRYOPRECIPITATE

Cryoprecipitate is derived from a single-donor blood donation unit (450 mL) that is concentrated by centrifugation to approximately 10 to 15 mL. The typical preparation is enriched in factor VIII, vWF, fibrinogen, fibronectin, and factor XIII. The major limitations of cryoprecipitate therapy are (1) the risk of viral transmission, because there are no viral inactivation steps in the manufacturing process; (2)

multiple units are required in order to provide the necessary replacement doses, resulting in large infusion volumes; and (3) thawing of cryoprecipitate preparations usually takes about 30 minutes.[21]

PROTHROMBIN COMPLEX CONCENTRATES

PCCs are intermediate-purity pooled plasma products containing a mixture of vitamin K–dependent proteins that are used for the treatment of hemophilia A and B. PCCs are produced by ion-exchange chromatography from the cryoprecipitate supernatant of large plasma pools after removal of antithrombin and factor XI.[22] Depending on the processing technique, either a 3-factor (eg, factors II, IX, and X) or 4-factor (eg, factors II, VII, IX, and X) concentrate contains a final overall clotting-factor concentration that is approximately 25 times higher than in normal plasma.[23] Most PCCs contain heparin in order to prevent activation of these factors. PCCs may also contain the coagulation inhibitors protein C and protein S. Two PCCs are currently available: Uman Complex D.I. (Kedrison, Castelvecchio Pascoli, Italy) and Prothromplex TIM 3 (Baxter, Vienna, Austria).[24] Both contain clotting factors II, IX, and X. In the United States, Kcentra gained FDA approval on April 30, 2013. It contains factors II, VII, IX, and X.

PCCs were originally indicated for the treatment of patients with hemophilia B. More recently, their indication has expanded as a replacement therapy for congenital or acquired deficiency of vitamin K–dependent clotting factors. At present, the main indication of PCC is for the urgent reversal of overanticoagulation with warfarin. The goal of urgent warfarin reversal is to increase the levels of, or replace, vitamin K–dependent clotting factors.[25] Multiple studies have shown that PCCs are more effective and predictable at correcting INR than FFP.[23,26,27] In addition, smaller volumes of PCC are needed to reverse anticoagulation.[28] PCCs are also an important therapeutic modality when urgent reversal of anticoagulation is required. They are safe, predictable, and efficient.

FACTOR VIIA

Factor VIIa is a recombinant agent that is used in the treatment of patients with factor VII deficiency and in patients with hemophilia A or B who have inhibitors. The mechanism of action of this factor is not completely understood but it is thought to control hemostasis by increasing thrombin generation on activated platelets. In addition, factor VIIa activates thrombin-activatable fibrinolysis inhibitor, which acts to stabilize the clot by inhibition of fibrinolysis.[29]

After the initial approval of recombinant factor (rFactor) VIIa there was much enthusiasm for its use to control bleeding in major trauma, cardiovascular surgery, and intracranial bleeding.[30–33] A prospective randomized multicenter study in 2005 reported that, in major patients with trauma, factor VIIa decreased the numbers of RBC transfusions and the number of patients requiring massive transfusions (>20 units of RBCs), but there was no survival benefit.[34] Subsequently the CONTROL trial, the largest placebo-controlled multicenter study to evaluate the use of factor VIIa in patients with trauma, failed to show differences in mortality or organ failure between the two groups.[35] Because of the lack of supporting evidence, the use of factor VIIa in trauma is not recommended.

The role of factor VIIa in cardiac surgery is still not well defined and its use in orthopedic, vascular, obstetrics/gynecology, and urogenital surgery has been limited because of the significant lack of high-quality clinical trials. Although a randomized placebo-controlled trial of 399 patients with intracerebral hemorrhage showed that factor VIIa limited the hemorrhage, when this study was expanded to 821 patients this agent failed to improve mortality and disability at the 90-day evaluation.[36] Furthermore, a major risk of factor VIIa use is thrombosis, particularly in patients with preexisting cardiovascular disease when this agent is used in conjunction with antifibrinolytic inhibitors or PCC.[29] At present, the accepted indications for the use of rFactor VIIa are limited to hemophilia A and B with inhibitors, acquired hemophilia, and factor VII deficiency.

FACTOR XIII

Once a fibrin clot is formed via the coagulation cascade it must be stabilized in order to prevent premature fibrinolysis. The crosslinking of the alpha and beta chain fibrin monomers is catalyzed by factor XIII, a transglutaminase that links glutamic acid on one fibrin chain with lysine residues on an adjacent fibrin monomer. Inherited factor XIII deficiency is an autosomal recessive condition that manifests with soft tissue bleeds, hemarthrosis, intracranial bleeding, bleeding during surgery, and poor wound healing. Solubility of fibrin clots is increased in factor XIII deficiency, therefore incubating the clots with solubilizing agents can confirm the diagnosis. Before 2011, FFP or cryoprecipitate was used to treat this deficiency; however, plasma-derived factor XIII concentrate (Corifact, CSL Behring) is now available in the United States. Factor XIII concentrate is administered intravenously to a level of 5% to 20%. Dosing is recommended at 10 to 75 IU every 4 to 6 weeks because of the long half-life of this product (9–15 days). Because the risk of cerebral hemorrhage is high in patients with this deficiency, prophylactic treatment is recommended (lower doses). Patients with bleeding episodes or requiring surgery should receive higher doses of factor XIII concentrate.[30,37]

FACTOR VIII

Hemophilia A is an X-linked disorder that affects 1 in 10,000 men. The major clinical manifestations in this disease are arthropathy secondary to spontaneous bleeding into joints with a risk of mortality from hemorrhagic bleeds ranging from 20% to 50% of patients.[38] Replacement therapy for hemophilia A was first described in 1832 and continues to advance, providing decreased risk of infectious disease transmission and increased attainment of high plasma levels of deficient factor. Pool and Robinson's[39] observation that the insoluble precipitate that results from thawing frozen plasma contains high concentrations of factor VIII formed the basis for development of the use of factor concentrates in modern transfusional medicine. This development resulted in the use of cryoprecipitate when levels of factor VIII could be replaced to greater than 20% in patients with hemophilia A.[39]

Plasma-derived factor concentrates first became available in the 1970s. Although drastically improving the life expectancy of hemophiliac patients, these agents almost uniformly transmitted several viral diseases, including hepatitis B and C as well as HIV. The safety of plasma-derived concentrates continues to improve and current viral inactivation practices (including solvent detergent, pasteurization, and nanofiltration) seem to have eradicated the transmission of hepatitis B, hepatitis C, and HIV. The currently available plasma-derived concentrates are classified as high purity (containing only the desired factor) or intermediate purity (containing the desired factor as well as other factors). Factor VIII intermediate-purity concentrates (Alphanate, Humate, Wilate) contain vWF. Intermediate-purity factor VIII concentrates are purified from cryoprecipitated plasma or FFP. Most of these products are stabilized with human albumin.[38]

rFactor VIII concentrates have been available since the 1990s. The currently available preparations are full-length factor VIII or B domain deleted (which is not required for coagulation activity). The recombinant protein is produced either in Chinese hamster ovary or baby hamster kidney cells. The first-generation recombinant product has human albumin added as a stabilizer, whereas the second generation of rFactor VIII (Kogenate) is stabilized with nonprotein additives. The third generation of rFactor VIII concentrates (Advate, Xyntha) are devoid of human products, making these factor replacements the safest with regard to disease transmission as well as providing unlimited availability.[38]

Factor VIII replacement therapy in hemophilia A depends on the type of surgery or bleeding event. For minor surgery, including dental extractions, a desired level of factor VIII replacement (20 U/kg) is greater than 30%, whereas replacement in the trauma or major surgical setting requires levels of 100%. In general, the administration of 1 U of factor VIII concentrate increases the level by 2%. Factor VIII therapy is continued for 1 to 3 days postoperatively for minor procedures; however, 50% replacement for 10 to 14 days is usually required for major bleeds. Dosing is usually accomplished in bolus infusions every 8 to 12 hours with continuous monitoring of factor levels.[40]

One of the major complications of treating patients with hemophilia A is the development of antibodies to factor VIII. However, this problem is seen in approximately 30% of patients and often develops early after the initiation of replacement therapy. In patients with low titer levels of inhibitors, increasing the dose of factor VIII usually suffices in achieving adequate hemostasis. In patients with high levels of titer inhibitors or individuals with low levels of titer inhibitors who fail to respond to increased factor VIII doses, bypass therapy using agents that activate the coagulation pathway beyond factor VIIIa may be necessary. At present, the available bypass agents include PCC and recombinant factor VIIa. However, both of these agents carry an increased risk of thrombosis.[40]

FACTOR IX

Hemophilia B or Christmas disease is an X-linked disorder that affects 1 in 30,000 people. The clinical course and morbidity of hemophilia B are similar to those seen in hemophilia A. One notable exception is that the development of inhibitors is much less common in hemophilia B. Three replacement therapies are presently available for the treatment of factor IX deficiency:

1. Factor IX complex (Bebulin, Profilnine), also called PCC
2. Coagulation factor IX concentrate (Mononine, AlphaNine SD), a high-purity plasma-derived product
3. Recombinant factor IX concentrate (BeneFix), a nanofiltered product that is produced without animal or human proteins

In patients with hemophilia B undergoing minor surgical procedures, such as dental extractions or implant placement, the recommended replacement of factor IX is greater than 30% (40 U/kg). Patients with major bleeds, trauma, or requiring major surgical procedures should be replaced to 100% (125 U/kg) and maintained throughout the postoperative period at a level of 50% or greater. Patients with high titer factor IX inhibitors should be treated with bypass therapy (PCC or factor VIIa) as described earlier.[38,40]

ANTI-INHIBITOR COAGULANT COMPLEX

After exposure to factor VIII, alloantibodies (inhibitors) that neutralize factor VIII clotting function develop in approximately 30% of patients with severe hemophilia A.[41] The development of high titer factor VIII inhibitors complicates treatment because bleeding no longer responds to standard factor VIII replacement.[42] Alternative forms of clotting-factor concentrates, known as bypassing agents, are used to treat bleeding in these patients. Two of these agents are anti-inhibitor coagulant complex (AICC) and recombinant factor VIIa. Both agents control approximately 80% of bleeding episodes in patients with hemophilia and inhibitors. AICC is used to control bleeding episodes or bleeding during surgery in patients with hemophilia A and hemophilia B. It contains coagulation factors (eg, nonactivated factors II, IX, and X; and factor VIIa) that are normally produced in the body.

Many studies have shown the safety of AICC. Leissinger and colleagues[43] showed that AICC prophylaxis at a dose of 85 U/kg ($\pm$15%), administered on 3 nonconsecutive days weekly, significantly decreased overall bleeding, hemarthroses, and target-joint bleeding and was associated with few adverse effects in patients with hemophilia A. Hilgartner and Knatterud[44] conducted a multicenter study that evaluated the efficacy of AICC in the treatment of joint, mucous membrane, musculocutaneous, and emergency bleeding episodes such as central nervous system hemorrhages and surgical bleedings. Of the 49 patients enrolled in the study, 44 patients had a diagnosis of hemophilia A with inhibitors, 3 patients had a diagnosis of hemophilia B with inhibitors, and 2 patients were diagnosed with acquired factor VIII inhibitor. Forty-nine patients with inhibitor titers greater than 5 Bethesda units were given 489 single doses for the treatment of 165 bleeding episodes. The usual dose was 50 Units per kilogram of body weight, which was repeated at 12-hour intervals (6-hour intervals in mucous membrane bleedings), if necessary. The researchers reported that bleeding was controlled in 153 episodes (93%), and in 130 (78%) of the episodes hemostasis was achieved with 1 or more infusions within 36 hours (36% were controlled with 1 infusion within 12 hours). An additional 14% of episodes responded after more than 36 hours. Of the 489 single doses administered, 3.7% caused minor transient reactions in the recipients. Researchers reported that 10 patients (20%) showed an increase in their inhibitor titers, and in 5 of those patients (10%) the increase was 10-fold or more. The researchers concluded that AICC seems to be safe and efficacious in the treatment of bleeding episodes with factor VIII or factor IX deficiencies with inhibitors.[44]

FIBRINOGEN CONCENTRATE

Fibrinogen concentrate is indicated for the treatment of acute bleeding episodes in patients with congenital fibrinogen deficiency, including afibrinogenemia and hypofibrinogenemia. It is also used as secondary prophylaxis in cases in which there has been potentially life-threatening bleeding at high risk of recurrence (eg, intracranial hemorrhage).[45] It is produced from pooled human plasma using the Cohn/Oncley cryoprecipitation procedure.[46] The concentration of fibrinogen is standardized; the product is stored as a lyophilized powder at room temperature and can be reconstituted quickly with sterile water, and infusion volumes are low, allowing rapid administration without delays for thawing or crossmatching.[47]

Four fibrinogen concentrates are currently available: Haemocomplettan (CSL Behring, Marburg, Germany), FIBRINOGENE T1 and Clottagen (LFB, Les Ulis, France), Fibrinogen HT (Benesis, Osaka, Japan), and FibroRAAS (Shanghai RAAS, Shanghai, China).[48,49] However, the most widely used is Haemocomplettan (commercialized in the United States as RiaSTAP).[50] RiaSTAP is a human pasteurized, highly purified, plasma-derived fibrinogen concentrate.

Several preclinical studies show that substitution therapy with fibrinogen concentrate may reverse a dilutional coagulopathy by replacing the missing factor and restoring fibrin production and clot formation.[51] In addition, retrospective clinical analyses suggest a potential hemostatic effect of substitution therapy with fibrinogen concentrate in bleeding patients. Fibrinogen concentrate also significantly improves whole-blood clot firmness and reduces the postoperative transfusion requirements in severely bleeding patients.[47,51] The median postinfusion fibrinogen levels were 1.45 g/L and reductions in both thrombin and activated partial thromboplastin time were observed after infusion. The median single and total doses per episode were 2.0 and 4.0 g per patient, respectively, and the median duration of treatment was 1 day.[50] In a prospective clinical study of orthopedic patients receiving volume replacement, fibrinogen concentrate restored clotting function, reversing the effects of dilutional coagulopathy.[22]

FACTOR XIII-A SUBUNIT

Factor XIII-A subunit is a recombinant human factor XIII-A2 homodimer composed of 2 factor XIII-A subunits. The factor XIII-A subunit is a 731 amino acid chain with an acetylated N-terminal serine. When factor XIII is activated by thrombin, a 37-amino-acid peptide is cleaved from the N-terminus of the A subunit.[52] In the United States, Tretten, recombinant factor XIII-A subunit, was FDA approved on December 23, 2013 as the first recombinant product for use in the routine prevention of bleeding in adults and children who have congenital factor XIII-A subunit deficiency.[53]

Tretten is supplied as a sterile, white, lyophilized powder in a single-use vial. After reconstitution with 3.2 mL of sterile water for injection, each vial contains 667 to 1042 IU/mL of recombinant coagulation factor XIII-A subunit. The reconstituted solution has a pH of approximately 8.0. The formulation contains no preservative and must only be administered intravenously.[52] The dose for routine prophylaxis for bleeding in patients with congenital factor XIII-A subunit deficiency is 35 IU per kilogram of body weight once monthly to achieve a target trough level of FXIII activity at or greater than 10% using a validated assay.[54]

TRANSFUSION COMPLICATIONS

Acute transfusion reactions are rare. They usually occur at 0.24% of transfusions.[55] Acute transfusion reactions usually present during or within 24 hours of a blood transfusion. The most frequent reactions include fever, chills, pruritus, or urticaria, which typically resolve promptly without specific treatment or complications. Other signs include severe shortness of breath, red urine, high fever, or loss of consciousness, which might be the first indication of a more severe and potentially fatal reaction.[55]

Acute transfusion reactions are typically classified into the following entities[56]:

- Volume overload
- Bacterial contamination and endotoxemia
- Acute hemolytic reactions
- Nonhemolytic febrile reactions
- TRALI
- Allergic reactions

Volume Overload

Volume overload occurs when the volume of the transfused blood components and that of any coincidental infusions cause acute hypervolemia, which can lead to acute pulmonary edema.[57]

Bacterial Contamination and Endotoxemia

Bacterial contamination and endotoxemia may result from any of the following:

- Opening the blood container in a nonsterile environment
- Inadequate sterile preparation of the phlebotomy site
- The presence of bacteria in the donor's circulation at the time of blood collection

Acute Hemolytic Reactions

Acute hemolytic reactions may be either immune mediated or non–immune mediated. Immune-mediated hemolytic transfusion reactions are usually caused by immunoglobulin (Ig) M (anti-A, anti-B, or anti-A, B). They result in severe and potentially fatal complement-mediated intravascular hemolysis. Immune-mediated hemolytic reactions caused by IgG, Rh, Kell, Duffy, or other non-ABO antibodies typically result in extravascular sequestration, shortened survival of transfused red cells, and mild clinical reactions.[58]

Nonimmune hemolytic transfusion reactions occur when RBCs are damaged before transfusion, resulting in hemoglobinemia and hemoglobinuria without significant clinical symptoms.[59]

Nonhemolytic Febrile Reactions

Nonhemolytic febrile reactions are usually caused by cytokines from leukocytes in transfused red cell or platelet components. This condition results in fever, chills, or rigors. A nonhemolytic transfusion reaction is a diagnosis of exclusion because hemolytic and septic reactions can present similarly.

Transfusion-Related Acute Lung Injury

TRALI has 2 proposed pathophysiologic mechanisms: the antibody hypothesis and the neutrophil priming hypothesis. Both mechanisms lead to pulmonary edema in the absence of circulatory overload.[60,61]

The antibody hypothesis states that an HLA class I, HLA class II, or human neutrophil antigen antibody in the transfused component reacts with neutrophil antigens in the recipient. The recipient's neutrophils lodge in the pulmonary capillaries and release mediators that cause pulmonary capillary leakage. As a consequence, many patients with TRALI develop transient leukopenia. The neutrophil priming hypothesis does not require antigen-antibody interactions and occurs in patients with clinical conditions that predispose to neutrophil priming and endothelial activation, such as infection, surgery, or inflammation. Bioactive substances in the transfused component activate the primed, sequestered neutrophils, and pulmonary endothelial damage occurs.

Allergic Reactions

Allergic reactions present with rash, urticaria, or pruritus. They are usually IgE mediated. These reactions are attributed to hypersensitivity to soluble allergens found in the transfused blood component.[62,63]

SUMMARY

Blood products are routinely used to manage various coagulation and hematological disorders. Oral and maxillofacial surgeons must have a basic knowledge and understanding of the various available products. A consultation with each patient's hematologist is always advised in order to decrease the risk of adverse events and improve the patient's safety.

REFERENCES

1. Heébert PC, Wells G, Blajchman MA, et al. A multicenter, randomized, controlled clinical trial of transfusion requirements in critical care. Transfusion Requirements in Critical Care Investigators, Canadian Critical Care Trials Group. N Engl J Med 1999;340(6):409–17.
2. Lacroix J, Heébert PC, Hutchison JS, et al. Transfusion strategies for patients in pediatric intensive care units. N Engl J Med 2007;356(16):1609–19.
3. King KE, Bandarenko N. Blood transfusion therapy: a physician's hand- book. 9th edition. Bethesda (MD): American Association of Blood Banks; 2008. p. 236.
4. Klein HG, Spahn DR, Carson JL. Red blood cell transfusion in clinical practice. Lancet 2007;370(9585):415–26.
5. Carless PA, Henry DA, Carson JL, et al. Transfusion thresholds and other strategies for guiding allogeneic red blood cell transfusion. Cochrane Database Syst Rev 2010;(10):CD002042.
6. Carson TH, editor. Standards for blood banks and transfusion services. 27th edition. Bethesda (MD): AABB; 2011.
7. Whitaker BI. The 2007 nationwide blood collection and utilization survey report. Bethesda (MD): AABB; 2007.
8. Ness P, Braine H, King K, et al. Single-donor platelets reduce the risk of septic platelet transfusion reactions. Transfusion 2001;41:857.
9. Kaufman RM. Chapter 113, principles of platelet transfusion therapy. In: Hoffman R, editor. Hematology: basic principles and practice. 6th edition. Philadelphia: Churchill Livingstone; 2013. p. 1653–58
10. Murphy S, Gardner FH. Effect of storage temperature on maintenance of platelet viability: deleterious effect of refrigerated storage. N Engl J Med 1969; 280:1094.
11. The Trial to Reduce Alloimmunization to Platelets Study Group. Leukocyte reduction and ultraviolet B irradiation of platelets to prevent alloimmunization and refractoriness to platelet transfusions. N Engl J Med 1997;337:1861.
12. Practice guidelines for blood component therapy: A report by the American Society of Anesthesiologists Task Force on Blood Component Therapy. Anesthesiology 1996;84:732.
13. Rebulla P. Platelet transfusion trigger in difficult patients. Transfus Clin Biol 2001;8:249.
14. Clark P, Mintz PD. Transfusion triggers for blood components. Curr Opin Hematol 2001;8:387.
15. Blumberg N, Heal JM, Phillips GL. Platelet transfusions: trigger, dose, benefits, and risks. F1000 Med Rep 2010;2:5.
16. Annen K, Olson JE. Optimizing platelet transfusions. Curr Opin Hematol 2015;22:559.
17. Karafin MS, Hillyer CD, Shaz BH. Chapter 116, principles of plasma transfusion: plasma, cryoprecipitate, albumin, and immunoglobulins. In: Hoffman R, editor. Hematology: basic principles and practice. 6th edition. Philadelphia: Churchill Livingstone; 2013. p. 1683–94.
18. Holcomb JB, del Junco DJ, Fox EE, et al. The Prospective, Observational, Multicenter, Major Trauma Transfusion (PROMMTT) study: comparative effectiveness of a time-varying treatment with competing risks. JAMA Surg 2013;148:127.
19. Holcomb JB, Shibani P. Optimal trauma resuscitation with plasma as the primary resuscitative fluid: the surgeon's perspective. Hematology Am Soc Hematol Educ Program 2013;2013:656.
20. Holcomb JB, Tilley BC, Baraniuk S, et al, PROPPR Study Group. Transfusion of plasma, platelets, and red blood cells in a 1:1:1 vs a 1:1:2 ratio and mortality in patients with severe trauma: the PROPPR randomized clinical trial. JAMA 2015;313:471.
21. Clark DB. Chapter 117, preparation of plasma-derived and recombinant human plasma proteins. In: Hoffman R, editor. Hematology: basic principles and practice. 6th edition. Philadelphia: Churchill Livingstone; 2013. p. 1695–1704.

22. Mittermayr M, Streif W, Haas T, et al. Hemostatic changes after crystalloid or colloid fluid administration during major orthopedic surgery: the role of fibrinogen administration. Anesth Analg 2007;105: 905–17.

23. Hellstern P. Production and composition of prothrombin complex concentrates: correlation between composition and therapeutic efficiency. Thromb Res 1999;95:S7–12.

24. Schuman S, Bijsterveld N. Anticoagulants and their reversal. Transfus Med Rev 2007;21:37–48.

25. Santagostino E, Mannucci PM. Guidelines on replacement therapy for haemophilia and inherited coagulation disorders in Italy. Haemophilia 2000;6: 1–10.

26. Makris M. Optimisation of the prothrombin complex concentrate dose for warfarin reversal. Thromb Res 2005;115:451–3.

27. Erber W, Perry D. Plasma and plasma products in the treatment of massive haemorrhage. Best Pract Res Clin Haematol 2006;19:97–112.

28. Makris M, Greaves M, Phillips W, et al. Emergency oral anticoagulant reversal: the relative efficacy of infusions of fresh frozen plasma and clotting factor concentrate on correction of the coagulopathy. Thromb Haemost 1997;77:477–80.

29. Reding MT, Key NS. Chapter 161, hematologic problems in the surgical patient: bleeding and thrombosis in immunoglobulins. In: Hoffman R, editor. Hematology: basic principles and practice. 6th edition. Philadelphia: Churchill Livingstone; 2013. p. 2234–51.

30. Gailani D, Neff AT. Chapter 139, rare coagulation factor deficiencies in immunoglobulins. In: Hoffman R, editor. Hematology: basic principles and practice. 6th edition. Philadelphia: Churchill Livingstone; 2013. p. 1971–86.

31. Logan AC, Yank V, Stafford RS. Off-label use of recombinant factor VIIa in U.S. hospitals: analysis of hospital records. Ann Intern Med 2011;154: 516.

32. Kenet G, Walden R, Eldad A, et al. Treatment of traumatic bleeding with recombinant factor VIIa. Lancet 1999;354:1879.

33. Boffard KD, Riou B, Warren B, et al. Recombinant factor VIIa as adjunctive therapy for bleeding control in severely injured trauma patients: two parallel randomized, placebo-controlled, double-blind clinical trials. J Trauma 2005;59:8.

34. Knudson MM, Cohen MJ, Reidy R, et al. Trauma, transfusions, and use of recombinant factor VIIa: a multicenter case registry report of 380 patients from the Western Trauma Association. J Am Coll Surg 2011;212:87.

35. Dutton RP, Parr M, Tortella BJ, et al. Recombinant activated factor VII safety in trauma patients: results from the CONTROL trial. J Trauma 2011;71:12.

36. Mayer SA, Brun NC, Begtrup K, et al. Recombinant activated factor VII for acute intracerebral hemorrhage. N Engl J Med 2005;352:777.

37. What are rare clotting factor deficiencies? World Federation of Hemophilia (WFH), Montréal, CANADA, E-mail: wfh@wfh.org, 2009. Available at: http://www1.wfh.org/publication/files/pdf-1337.pdf.

38. Roman E, Larson PJ, Manno CS. Chapter 118, transfusion therapy for coagulation factor deficiencies. In: Hoffman R, editor. Hematology: basic principles and practice. 6th edition. Philadelphia: Churchill Livingstone; 2013. p. 1705–15.

39. Pool JG, Robinson J. Observations on plasma banking and transfusion procedures for haemophilic patients using a quantitative assay for antihaemophilic globulin (AHG). Br J Haematol 1959;5:24.

40. Carcao M, Moorehead P, Lillicrap D. Chapter 137, hemophilia A and B. In: Hoffman R, editor. Hematology: basic principles and practice. 6th edition. Philadelphia: Churchill Livingstone; 2013. p. 1940–60.

41. DiMichele D. Inhibitors: resolving diagnostic and therapeutic dilemmas. Haemophilia 2002;8:280–7.

42. Leissinger CA. Prevention of bleeds in hemophilia patients with inhibitors: emerging data and clinical direction. Am J Hematol 2004;77:187–93.

43. Leissinger C, Gringeri A, Antmen B, et al. Anti-inhibitor coagulant complex prophylaxis in hemophilia with inhibitors. N Engl J Med 2011;365:1684–92.

44. Hilgartner M, Knatterud G. The use of factor eight inhibitor by-passing activity (FEIBA immuno) product for treatment of bleeding episodes in hemophiliacs with inhibitors. Blood 1983;61(1):36–40.

45. Bolton-Maggs PH, Perry DJ, Chalmers EA, et al. The rare coagulation disorders–review with guidelines for management from the United Kingdom Haemophilia Centre Doctors' Organisation. Haemophilia 2004;10:593–628.

46. Rahe-Meyer N, Sørensen B. Fibrinogen concentrate for management of bleeding. J Thromb Haemost 2011;9:1–5.

47. Fenger-Eriksen C, Ingerslev J, Sorensen B. Fibrinogen concentrate–a potential universal hemostatic agent. Expert Opin Biol Ther 2009;9(10):1325–33.

48. Negrier C, Rothschild C, Goudemand J, et al. Pharmacokinetics and pharmacodynamics of a new highly secured fibrinogen concentrate. J Thromb Haemost 2008;6:1494–9.

49. Kreuz W, Meili E, Peter-Salonen K, et al. Pharmacokinetic properties of a pasteurised fibrinogen concentrate. Transfus Apher Sci 2005;32:239–46.

50. Kreuz W, Meili E, Peter-Salonen K, et al. Efficacy and tolerability of a pasteurised human fibrinogen concentrate in patients with congenital fibrinogen deficiency. Transfus Apher Sci 2005;32:247–53.

51. Fenger-Eriksen C, Jensen TM, Kristensen BS, et al. Fibrinogen substitution improves whole blood clot firmness after dilution with hydroxyethyl starch in

bleeding patients undergoing radical cystectomy: a randomized, placebo-controlled clinical trial. J Thromb Haemost 2009;7(5):795–802.

52. Tretten Web site. Available at: http://www.tretten-us.com. Accessed April 5, 2016.

53. US Food and Drug Administration FDA approves Tretten to treat rare genetic clotting disorder. Available at: http://www.fda.gov/NewsEvents/Newsroom/PressAnnouncements/ucm379696.htm. Accessed April 5, 2016.

54. Tretten: Highlights of prescribing information. Available at: http://www.fda.gov/downloads/BiologicsBlood Vaccines/BloodBloodProducts/ApprovedProducts/LicensedProductsBLAs/FractionatedPlasmaProducts/UCM379763.pdf. Accessed April 5, 2016.

55. Squires JE. Risks of transfusion. South Med J 2011; 104(11):762–9.

56. Keller-Stanislawski B, Lohmann A, Günay S, et al. The German Haemovigilance System–reports of serious adverse transfusion reactions between 1997 and 2007. Transfus Med 2009;19(6):340–9.

57. Rana R, Fernandez-Perez ER, Khan SA, et al. Transfusion-related acute lung injury and pulmonary edema in critically ill patients: a retrospective study. Transfusion 2006;46(9):1478–83.

58. Ness P, Creer M, Rodgers GM, et al. Building an immune-mediated coagulopathy consensus: early recognition and evaluation to enhance post-surgical patient safety. Patient Saf Surg 2009;3(1):8.

59. Sandler SG, Berry E, Ziotnick A. Benign hemoglobinuria following transfusion of accidentally frozen blood. JAMA 1976;235(26):2850–1.

60. Silliman CC. The two-event model of transfusion-related acute lung injury. Crit Care Med 2006;34(5 Suppl):S124–31.

61. Silliman CC, Curtis BR, Kopko PM, et al. Donor antibodies to HNA-3a implicated in TRALI reactions prime neutrophils and cause PMN-mediated damage to human pulmonary microvascular endothelial cells in a two-event in vitro model. Blood 2007; 109(4):1752–5.

62. Vamvakas EC, Pineda AA. Allergic and anaphylactic reactions. In: Popovsky MA, editor. Transfusion reactions. 2nd edition. Bethesda (MD): American Association of Blood Banks Press; 2001. p. 83–127.

63. The 2011 National Blood Collection and Utilization Survey Report. Report of the US Department of Health and Human Services. Available at: http://www.hhs.gov/ash/bloodsafety/2011-nbcus.pdf. Accessed April 5, 2016.

Damage Control Resuscitation for Catastrophic Bleeding

 CrossMark

Chase L. Andreason, DMD[a],
Timothy H. Pohlman, MD, FACS[b],*

KEYWORDS

- Hemorrhage • Shock • Transfusion • Resuscitation • Coagulopathy • Thrombelastography

KEY POINTS

- The timely recognition of shock secondary to hemorrhage from severe facial trauma or as a complication of complex oral and maxillofacial surgery presents formidable challenges clinically.
- Specific hemostatic disorders are induced by hemorrhage and several extreme homeostatic imbalances may appear during, or in the aftermath of, resuscitation of patients with catastrophic bleeding that dominate the pathophysiology of an acutely bleeding patient.
- Damage control resuscitation (DCR) has evolved from a definition of massive transfusion (MT) to a more complex therapeutic paradigm that includes hemodynamic resuscitation, hemostatic resuscitation, and homeostatic resuscitation.
- A detailed DCR protocol must be and should be an essential element of a well-defined response to catastrophic blood loss that may complicate several surgical and medical specialties.
- In virtually every clinical setting, however, definitive control of bleeding is the principal objective of any comprehensive resuscitation scheme for hemorrhagic shock (HS), and DCR should not overshadow emergent intervention to that end.

INTRODUCTION

In the past decade, MT for exsanguinating hemorrhage has evolved into a more inclusive paradigm referred to as DCR. DCR centers on 3 distinct therapeutic objectives: hemodynamic resuscitation, hemostatic resuscitation, and homeostatic resuscitation. The principles of DCR are based on extensive laboratory investigation and comprehensive clinical study of HS pathophysiology, hemorrhage-associated coagulopathy, and hemorrhage-induced homeostatic imbalance, which appear as a consequence of massive blood loss or in the aftermath of resuscitation.[1–7] Implementation of team-based DCR programs is associated with an increase in survival of the severely injured in concert with a reduction in costly waste of blood bank products.[8,9] Blood component transfusion best practices were developed by the AABB to enhance outcome measures of hospital blood management programs,[10] and, currently, hospitals in the United States are required by accreditation and regulatory agencies[a] to institute specific resuscitation policies and guidelines. Moreover, trauma center verification by the American College of Surgeons Committee on Trauma

[a] Department of Oral Surgery and Hospital Dentistry, Indiana University School of Dentistry, 1121 West Michigan Street, Indianapolis, IN 46202, USA; [b] Trauma Services, Division of General Surgery, Department of Surgery, Methodist Hospital, Indiana University Health, Suite B238, 1701 North Senate Boulevard, Indianapolis, IN 46202, USA
* Corresponding author.
E-mail address: tpohlman@iuhealth.org

[a]The National Quality Measures Clearinghouse, sponsored by the Agency for Healthcare Research and Quality, and the US Department of Health and Human Services, have included The Joint Commission measures in its public database for evidence-based quality measures and measure sets.

Oral Maxillofacial Surg Clin N Am 28 (2016) 553–568
http://dx.doi.org/10.1016/j.coms.2016.06.010

oralmaxsurgery.theclinics.com

requires hospital to demonstrate both organized capability to carry out DCR and a commitment to the process.[11] DCR, however, is demanding with respect to resource utilization prompting considerable discourse and ethical debate on, for example, blood resource allocation in MT scenarios that create significant blood product shortages. Also at issue are the inherent exigencies of an emergency setting that compromise determination of futility, obtaining informed consent, and awareness of advanced directives.[12]

This article reviews the essential elements of DCR and describes application of this complex therapy to catastrophic bleeding in severely injured patients. Furthermore, the authors believe that the basic tenets of DCR elucidated in this review pertain to management of significant blood loss as a complication of complex oral and maxillofacial surgery as well as other conditions, for example, massive gastrointestinal bleeding, gynecologic hemorrhagic crises, and intraoperative and postoperative hemorrhage complicating vascular or cardiovascular procedures. Thus, clinicians of varying specialties must maintain familiarity with rapid and significant developments in this aspect of resuscitation. However, DCR is not the definitive management of life-threatening hemorrhage in most cases. The primary treatment of ongoing hemorrhage remains source control by surgical, angiographic, or endoscopic intervention.

HEMORRHAGIC SHOCK
Clinical Aspects

The early recognition of HS and timely initiation of resuscitation remain formidable challenges,[13] in part because of a complex mosaic of compensatory mechanisms activated in response to an acute loss of blood. Compensatory physiology tends to obscure signs of tissue hypoperfusion and impending hemodynamic collapse. Consequently, a substantial loss of blood sustained by a trauma patient prior to hospital arrival may pass unnoticed, or occult hemorrhage that continues in the trauma bay may not be recognized in a timely manner. In a previously healthy patient, these early compensatory processes are highly effective and create a deceptive clinical state that may suggest stability when rather a considerable oxygen debt has accumulated and significant cellular dysfunction has developed.[14]

Compensatory mechanisms are mediated by an increase in sympathetic autonomic activity in conjunction with secretion of vasoactive hormones (predominantly catecholamines, vasopressin, and angiotensin[15]) that mitigate the

reduction in perfusion of vital organs despite a fall in circulating blood volume. Decompensation generally means that the limits of these particular responses have been exceeded. Thus, under intense neurohormonal stimulation, an initial clinical state of compensated shock develops. Ongoing hemorrhage eventually progresses, however, to decompensated shock, characterized by hemodynamic instability and accelerating functional deterioration in vital physiologic systems,[16] and finally to refractory shock (also referred to as irreversible shock), associated with hemodynamic collapse and death.[17,18] Resuscitation initiated promptly and guided by established standards of care generally is effective for compensated HS. Resuscitation becomes progressively less effective during the decompensated phase of shock as physiologic reserves are exhausted and is rendered completely ineffective during the refractory phase due to accumulated cell death preventing recovery of organ function.

Because HS is fundamentally a problem of blood flow rather than blood pressure, systemic arterial hypotension (systolic blood pressure [SBP] $\leq$90 mm Hg) is widely regarded as an inaccurate clinical indicator of shock.[19–23] A change in heart rate (HR) assessed out of context with other parameters is also considered an insensitive as well as nonspecific sign of hemorrhage.[24] The ratio of HR to SBP, or shock index (SI), however, has been examined as a clinical measure that may identify hypoperfusion before a patient decompensates.[25–30] Furthermore, age diminishes physiologic reserve, and the product of SI and age is suggested as a more sensitive indicator compared with HR, SBP, or SI alone.[28] A yet more sensitive indication of occult hemorrhage may be obtained by dividing HR by the pulse pressure (SBP − diastolic blood pressure), referred to as the pulse rate over pressure evaluation (ROPE) index.[31] The ROPE index may be somewhat more sensitive to blood loss than SI.[32] A reduction in pulse pressure (also referred to as narrowing) reflects a downward trend in SBP due to diminished stroke volume in parallel with an upward trend in DBP due to compensatory vasoconstriction and an increase in vascular resistance.

Detection of a lactic acidosis corroborates the diagnosis of HS. A normal hydrogen ion (H^+) concentration ($[H^+]$) in extracellular fluid is 40 nmol/L, approximately one-millionth the extracellular concentration of HCO_3^- (normal, 24 mmol/L). Thus, the rise in $[H^+]$ secondary to a hemorrhage-induced acidemia is very small. For example, a substantial decrease in pH from 7.4 to 7.1 represents merely a 40-nmol/L increase in $[H^+]$. In addition to pH, this extraordinarily small number can be indirectly expressed as the amount of base that must be added to an acidotic patient to restore blood and extracellular fluid pH to 7.4. This quantity is referred to as base excess (BE), and by convention a BE value proceeded by a negative sign indicates acidosis requiring addition of base.[33] Exogenously administered bicarbonate effects the determination of BE and prevents the utilization of sequential determinations of this important measure in therapeutic decisions.[33] Ethanol intoxication decreases BE in trauma patients but in general does not confound identification of patients who are severely injured.[34]

Hemorrhage-associated Coagulopathy

Specific hemostatic defects appear prior to initiation of resuscitation in approximately 25% of severely injured patients[35–37] (**Fig. 1**). Trauma-associated coagulopathy (TAC) is an independent predictor of adverse outcomes and has been shown to lead to the prolongation of ICU and hospital lengths of stay and a 4-fold increase in mortality.[38] Trauma-induced modification of endothelial cell function has been examined as the principal mechanism of TAC.[39–43] TAC is considered part of a diffuse endotheliopathy model of systemic disturbance that is postulated to develop as a consequences of trauma and severe hemorrhage. In addition to TAC, a trauma-induced or hemorrhage-induced endotheliopathy is hypothesized to underlie disturbances of inflammation, blood-organ endothelial barrier integrity, and vasoregulation, which cause vascular leak, tissue edema, microvascular thrombi, diminished organ perfusion, uncontrolled hemorrhage, and organ injury.[5]

TAC likely involves enhanced expression of endothelial surface receptors for protein C and thrombomodulin (TM).[44] TM binds thrombin and converts the substrate specificity of thrombin to protein C. Up-regulation of these 2 endothelial cell receptors together accelerates the conversion of protein C to activated protein C (aPC),[45] and in the presence of protein S, increases aPC-mediated inhibition of activated coagulation factor (FV) IIIa and FVa,[46] thereby reducing the activity of FIXa and FXa, respectively. Disruption of the glycocalyx overlying the luminal surface of the endothelium is also observed. Damaged endothelial glycocalyx releases negatively charged proteoglycans, glycoproteins, glycolipids, and other heparin-like molecules,[47] which, in effect, heparinize a bleeding trauma patient.[48] Other mechanisms attributed to TAC include an acquired defect in platelet function (in particular impaired ADP-mediated platelet aggregation associated with traumatic brain injury),[49,50] depletion of coagulation factors and platelets lost through hemorrhage and deposition into injured tissue,[51] and consumption of platelets and coagulation factors secondary to disseminated intravascular coagulation[52] or to hyperfibrinolysis.[53]

Fibrinolysis is required as part of normal hemostasis. A physiologic release of endogenous tPA in response to trauma is thought to be essential

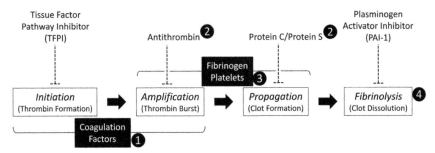

Fig. 1. Hemostasis and TAC. In response to injury, coagulation occurs in 3 distinct but overlapping phases: initiation, during which small amounts of coagulation factors are activated, notably FIX and FX, by tissue factor in the presence of FVIIa; amplification (alternatively referred to as priming), in which FXa produces a small amount of thrombin insufficient to cleave fibrinogen but adequate to activate FVIII, FV, and platelets; and propagation, by which activated coagulation factors assemble on aggregating platelets and produce a so-called thrombin burst in amounts that can convert fibrinogen to fibrin. Normal clot maturation also depends on a certain level of fibrinolysis after the conversion of plasminogen to plasmin by tPA, released from endothelium. Each phase is associated with an inhibitor or inhibitors, examples of which are shown connected by dotted lines. The proposed mechanisms of TAC include (1) depletion of coagulation factors; (2) endothelial cell injury with release of heparin-like proteoglycans that bind to antithrombin inhibiting coagulation factor activity and up-regulation of TM and endothelial receptor for protein C that converts protein C to aPC (which inhibits coagulation by blocking FVa and FVIIIa), (3) a qualitative defect I platelet function (especially in traumatic brain injury), and (4) consumption of coagulation factors, including fibrinogen substrate due to hyperfibrinolysis or disseminated intravascular coagulation.

to prevent propagation of the clotting process beyond sites of injury.[54] In particular, control of coagulation by fibrinolysis is thought to avert intravascular thrombosis in microvascular circuits. Disruption of microvascular perfusion, if extensive, may precipitate organ failure. The exact physiologic function of fibrinolysis in clot formation is made less clear, however, by the observation that neither congenital plasminogen deficiency nor congenital dysplasminogenemia is causally linked to any thromboembolic phenomena.[55,56]

The incidence of hyperfibrinolysis in severely injured patients has been reported to be 2% to 20%, which may increase to an incidence of 53% in patients who progress and require DCR.[57] Hemodilution during resuscitation in conjunction with a decrease in endogenous antifibrinolytic proteins, plasminogen activator inhibitor-1, α_2-antiplasmin, and thrombin-activatable fibrinolysis inhibitor can contribute to acquisition of hyperfibrinolysis as a complication of severe injury.[58] In addition, Moore and colleagues,[59] using thromboelastography, have identified a second acquired fibrinolytic phenotype occurring as a systemic manifestation of severe injury and referred to as fibrinolysis shutdown. Fibrinolysis shutdown is recognized as a relative resistance to tPA caused by trauma-induced dysregulation of plasmin formation. Both fibrinolysis shutdown and hyperfibrinolysis are associated with an increase in morbidity and mortality compared with patients with similar severity of injury but normal fibrinolysis physiology. Fulminate hyperfibrinolysis occurs in a small percentage of trauma patients, which is indicated by a characteristic diamond-shaped TEG tracing (**Fig. 2**). This specific coagulopathy is associated with a clinical state that is considered nonsurvivable.[60]

Fibrin monomers and fibrinogen degradation products contribute to coagulopathy in hemorrhaging patients by interfering with fibrin polymerization, clot stabilization[61] and by blocking ADP-induced platelet aggregation.[62] A bleeding tendency due to this mechanism may be intensified in patients with preexisting liver disease or hypoxic injury to the liver (shock liver), due to decreased hepatic clearance of degradation products.[63]

DAMAGE CONTROL RESUSCITATION

DCR is most effective if guided by an established protocol, which in part decreases the time to onset of transfusion. This leads to reductions in organ failure and other postinjury complications associated with severe hemorrhage.[8,64,65] DCR protocols should identify clinical thresholds to initiate DCR for a bleeding patient based on one of several validated models that predict MT.[7] In addition, an effective DCR protocol specifies authority to activate, delineates responsibilities of members of the resuscitation team, and directs timing and kind of blood components that are transfused and suggest other products to consider for administration. Protocols also recommend clinical parameters to monitor and resuscitation endpoints to consider for discontinuation of DCR. Although in most centers resuscitation of this magnitude is a rare event, DCR can be expected to use a vastly disproportionate share of resources.[7]

Hemodynamic Resuscitation

The total amount of oxygen transported to the periphery (oxygen delivery [DO_2]), at rest, is approximately 1.0 L/min (525 mL/min/m^2 and 625 mL/min/m^2 for an adult male and female of average height and weight, respectively). DO_2 is reduced during an acute loss of blood by a decrease in cardiac output caused by a decrease in venous return. Because the right and left sides of the heart are in series, cardiac output from the left ventricle must always equal venous return to the right atrium; the oxygen carrying capacity of blood, determined predominantly by hemoglobin concentration is less affected, particularly if the amount of crystalloid infused is minimized. (For practical reasons, the negligible amount of additional oxygen dissolved in plasma is ignored.) As DO_2 progressively falls, the amount of oxygen extracted as a fraction of the amount delivered (oxygen extraction ratio [O_2ER]) increases. This adaptive mechanism is critical to preservation of nominal organ system function despite depleted cardiovascular reserve and reduced DO_2. The point at which no further increase in O_2ER can occur in response to a falling DO_2 is referred to as the anaerobic threshold. The anaerobic threshold corresponds to the initiation of lactate production and signifies the boundary between compensated and decompensated HS. Any DO_2 below this threshold, designated DO_{2crit}, limits cellular respiration and may be considered the proximate cause of HS-induced organ dysfunction. This important relationship between DO_2 and DO_{2crit} varies considerably from one organ system to the next; it can be significantly modified by several external factors (infusion of inotropic agents, for example), and DO_{2crit} is not a distinct threshold.[66] For these reasons, clinical assessment of DO_{2crit} is impractical.[67] A reduction in DO_2 to less than DO_{2crit}, however, establishes a conceptual framework for the basic pathophysiology of HS (**Fig. 3**). Moreover, it defines the critical therapeutic goal of hemodynamic

A

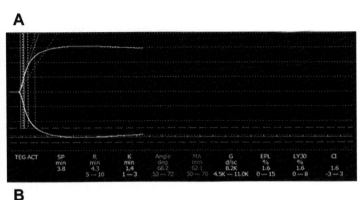

B

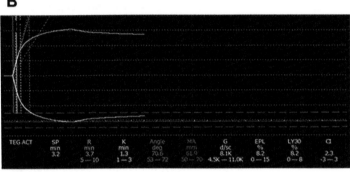

C

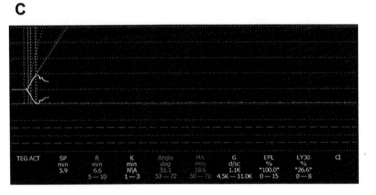

Fig. 2. TEG tracings for different fibrinolytic phenotypes. (A) Normal TEG tracing demonstrating normal clot kinetics and strength (adequate clotting factor activity, sufficient fibrinogen substrate, normal platelet function, normal platelet-fibrinogen interaction, and absence of abnormal fibrinolysis). (B) Abnormal TEG tracing demonstrating modest degree of secondary fibrinolysis (MA = 61.9 mm [normal 50–70 mm] and LY30 = 8.2% [normal 0%–8.0%]). (C) Abnormal TEG tracing demonstrating severe hyperfibrinolysis in a diamond-shape pattern suggesting nonsurvivability. TEG ACT, TEG activated clotting time.

resuscitation, which is to maximize tissue oxygenation. This can be achieved by restoration of adequate venous return while avoiding a significant dilution of oxygen carrying capacity through transfusion of packed red blood cells (RBCs), at times in massive amounts.

RBC transfusion is the critical component of hemodynamic resuscitation but may be compromised by an inexorable deterioration in biophysical and metabolic functions of erythrocytes stored at $4°C$ (for up to 42 days). These abnormalities are collectively referred to as a red cell storage lesion.[68] As an example, exhaustion of energy (ATP and ADP) during storage leads to depletion of 2,3-diphosphoglycerate (2,3-DPG) after approximately 21 days of RBC storage.[69,70] Binding of 2,3-DPG to hemoglobin decreases oxygen

affinity and promotes release of oxygen in the periphery. Depending on length of time in storage, RBCs transfused during DCR initially may not offload oxygen in sufficient amounts to meet cellular demand,[71] and the time required to regenerate 2,3-DPG in transfused RBCs in a recipient may exceed the brief time frame and extreme conditions of DCR. Methemoglobin, which also increases hemoglobin affinity for oxygen, accumulates in RBCs during storage[72] and may be incompletely reduced during DCR. Furthermore, the oxygen affinity of hemoglobin in transfused RBCs may be driven even higher by hypophosphatemia[73,74] and hypothermia, commonly encountered conditions in patients in HS. Thus a patient could potentially remain acidotic despite every indication of adequate perfusion and

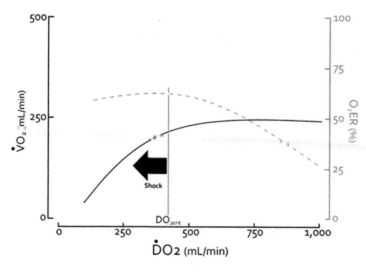

Fig. 3. DO_{2crit} defines shock. As DO_2 (*solid black line*) decreases secondary to a fall in cardiac output, drop in hemoglobin concentration, or both, O_2ER (*dashed line*) increases to maintain VO_2 constant ($Vo_2 = O_2ER \times DO_2$) until extraction is maximized. At this point, designated as DO_{2crit} (also referred to as the anaerobic threshold), VO_2 begins to decrease with further decreases in DO_2. When $DO_2 > DO_{2crit}$, VO_2 is flow-independent; when $DO_2 < DO_{2crit}$, VO_2 becomes flow-dependent. In addition, DO_{2crit} is associated with the onset of lactate formation and accumulation. Thus, shock can be defined conceptually as the presence of DO_2 less than DO_{2crit}, producing a reduction in VO_2. Normal $DO_2 = 800$ mL O_2/min-m^2; normal oxygen consumption (VO_2) = 200 mL O_2/min-m^2; normal $O_2ER = 25\%$.

transport of oxygen to the periphery after rapid replacement of 1 blood volume (10–12 U) in a short period of time.

In addition to these metabolic abnormalities, morphologic transformation in stored erythrocytes from flexible biconcave discs to rigid echinocytes (burr cells) and then to spheroechinocytes decreases microvascular flow due to obstruction of capillaries. RBC-mediated regulation of microvascular blood flow mediated by release of nitric oxide and ATP is abolished by storage.[75] This indirectly promotes a systemic proinflammatory state by triggering innate immune activation and by generating procoagulant bioactive phospholipids that are associated with an increased risk of acute lung injury.[76]

Whether transfusion of RBCs stored for shorter periods of time (<21 days) conveys an additional benefit by limiting adverse effects in the recipient remains controversial. Storage of RBCs, however, may be improved by cryopreservation at −80°C in a glycerol buffer solution to prevent membrane damage from ice crystal formation. Cryopreserved RBC transfusions are associated with improved transport of oxygen and an attenuated propensity for proinflammatory complications, including surgical site infection, transfusion-related acute lung injury (TRALI), multiple organ dysfunction syndrome, and multiple organ system failure.[77]

Hemostatic Resuscitation

Hemostatic resuscitation is achieved by transfusion of units of plasma and platelets in predetermined fixed amounts relative to the number of units of packed RBCs transfused. The intention

is to reconstitute the whole blood from which these components are derived. Instead of an empiric fixed ratio strategy, hemostatic resuscitation also can be goal directed by applying point-of-care (POC) viscoelastic coagulation testing. In practical terms, resuscitation may begin with an empiric dose of components and be followed by specific component transfusions based on determination of the patient's coagulation profile.

Fixed component ratio–directed damage control resuscitation

The efficacy of high component ratios was first identified in 2005 and was then referred to as balanced transfusion therapy.[78] Several clinical studies, largely retrospective in design, subsequently examined the MT of blood components (plasma, platelets, and RBCs) in different predetermined ratios. These studies have consistently indicated that survival improves significantly with higher ratios, that is, a higher number of units of plasma and platelets transfused relative to the number of units of packed RBCs transfused.[6,79–86] The empiric fixed ratio of units of plasma, platelets, and RBCs for DCR had been a matter of considerable controversy, with plasma:platelets:RBCs ratios between 1:1:3 and 1:1:1 suggested as optimal. Recently, this issue was examined in 12 level 1 trauma centers in the United States and Canada participating in the Pragmatic Randomized Optimal Platelet and Plasma Ratios trial, which prospectively examined 1:1:1 (high ratio) component transfusion compared with 1:1:2 (low ratio) component transfusion.[87] To participate, centers were required to have plasma available within 8 minutes of activating a DCR protocol. With survival as the primary endpoint, patients transfused with components in a high ratio were similar to patients transfused in a low ratio, which included patients who died of head trauma. Survival is significantly improved, however, in patients at risk for exsanguination in the immediate hours after injury if blood components are transfused in a high ratio (1:1:1) compared with patients transfused components at the low ratio (1:1:2). Furthermore, in the high ratio group, there was a significant reduction in the amount of plasma and other blood components transfused during resuscitation.[87]

A reduction in the time to first plasma transfusion during DCR significantly reduces mortality.[88] Stored thawed plasma, which contains acceptable coagulation factor activity for up to 5 days,[89] is the principal plasma component in most DCR protocols. AB plasma is transfused during DCR until a recipient's blood type can be determined. An empiric use of AB plasma may quickly exhaust a blood bank's supply of this limited resource. To minimize this problem, group A plasma has been used in DCR before blood type is known.[90–93] The risk of a blood group mismatch transfusion reaction is decreased by the fact that the most common encountered blood group in a recipient is group A, anti-B titers are generally low in donated group A plasma, and DCR patients typically receive several units of group O RBCs with plasma, which dilutes a potential target RBC antigen and decreases the risk of hemolysis due to ABO group mismatch.[91]

Bleeding-associated coagulopathy may occur secondary to the rapid development of hypofibrinogenemia.[94–96] Fibrinogen is depleted in the process of clot formation. Preexisting liver disease along with hypothermia may also diminish the synthesis of fibrinogen. Depletion of fibrinogen substrate can be exacerbated by an increase in plasmin-mediated degradation of any remaining fibrinogen if plasmin is in a high enough concentration (hyperfibrinogenolysis).[97] Also, acidosis, which frequently complicates DCR, accelerates plasmin-mediated fibrinogen degradation.[98] Four units of plasma deliver slightly under 2.5 g of fibrinogen (600 mg fibrinogen/U). If plasma is transfused early during DCR and continued at a high plasma:RBC ratio, sufficient amounts of fibrinogen should be transfused to obviate cryoprecipitate transfusion. In addition to fibrinogen, however, FXIII is enriched in cryoprecipitate. FXIII cross-links thrombin-generated fibrin strands and stabilizes forming clot, and this effect is not provided by plasma transfusion.

Goal-directed damage control resuscitation

Standard screening tests of coagulation, such as prothrombin time, activated partial thromboplastin time, and international normalized ratio, are performed on platelet-poor plasma at 37°C and do not reflect, for example, the important contribution of the cellular elements of blood to the formation of clot or the negative effect of hypothermia on coagulation.[99] Assessment of coagulation more applicable to DCR may include determination of the viscoelastic properties of a blood clot, such as clot strength and resistance to shear force (elasticity) and the presence of nonphysiologic fibrinolysis. Viscoelastic assays are most commonly performed by either thromboelastography (TEG) (Haemonetics Corp, Niles, IL, USA) (**Box 1**) or rotational thromboelastometry (ROTEM) (Tem International GmbH, Munich, Germany) in a clinical laboratory or as a POC coagulation test. At a basic level, each system determines essentially the same 5 viscoelastic parameters. These systems also estimate the rate and relative amount of thrombin generation, fibrinogen levels, platelet function, and degree of clot dissolution by fibrinolysis.[100] Thrombocytopenia may alter viscoelastic parameters significantly,[101] and consequently a platelet count should be included with a viscoelastic assessment of hemostasis. A resuscitation strategy that uses TEG or ROTEM as a more accurate (but still not perfect) assessment of hemostasis to determine what blood components to transfuse and the amount to transfuse as resuscitation progresses is referred to as goal-directed DCR.[102]

In the immediate onset of a DCR, POC viscoelastic coagulation tests do not provide critical data immediately and certainly not within time to inform decisions in a rapidly deteriorating clinical situation. Without a modification, data may not be provided any sooner than can be expected from laboratory screening tests.[103] In the TEG system, goal-directed resuscitation involves the use of rapid TEG (r-TEG) to diagnose and describe postinjury coagulopathy and to guide blood product replacement. For r-TEG, tissue factor is added with kaolin to activate coagulation, and recent data suggest that r-TEG can identify coagulation abnormalities very early after injury.[104] Blood products may be transfused in a fixed ratio initially for patients presenting with uncontrolled hemorrhage, with subsequent focused intervention based on r-TEG data, as they become available. Investigation with normal subjects suggests, however, that an r-TEG assay generates a clot that is more resistant to fibrinolysis initiated by tissue plasminogen activator (tPA) and that a thromboelastogram produced

---

Box 1
Basic viscoelastic parameters

Each TEG® parameter, R-time, K-time, α-angle, MA, and LY30, assess different components of hemostasis. Secondary, or derived quantities include G-value, and CI (or, coagulation index).

R-time: latency from time blood was placed in the TEG Analyzer until initial fibrin formation; represents enzymatic portion of coagulation.

   R-time prolonged: anticoagulants and factor deficiencies,

   R-time shortened: hypercoagulable states.

K-time: time to reach a clot strength of 20 mm of curve arm separation; represents *clot kinetics.*

   K-time shortened: increased fibrinogen level and, to a lesser extent, by platelet function,

   K-time prolonged: anticoagulants that affect both.

α-angle: rapidity (kinetics) of fibrin build-up and cross-linking, that is the speed of clot strengthening; represents fibrinogen level; α-angle is more comprehensive than K-time for this assessment.

   α-angle increased: increased fibrogen levels and, to a lesser extent, by platelet function,

   α angle decreased: anticoagulants that affect both.

   K-time and the α-angle provide similar information about the rate of clot buildup. Both are affected by availability of fibrinogen and by the presence or absence of coagulation factor XIII, which enables cross-linking of fibrin to form a stable clot; neither K-time, nor α-angle is influenced to any extent by platelets.

   K-time prolonged and α reduced: low fibrinogen level (factor XIII is rarely deficient)

MA: (maximum amplitude) direct function of the maximum dynamic properties of fibrin and platelet bonding; represents the ultimate strength of the fibrin clot. MA predominately reflects platelet function; MA also reflects fibrinogen availability and/or function to a lesser, but still important extent.

   MA is affected by platelet number and function and, to a lesser extent, by fibrinogen level. However, MA and both K-time and α-angle, are correlated due to the interaction between fibrinogen and platelets which through complex interactions produce the final clot.

LY30: measures the rate of amplitude reduction 30 minutes after MA. This reflects clot lysis and the ultimate stability of the clot. A LY30 greater than 3% represents hyperfibrinolysis and indicates an increased mortality risk.

G-value: expresses the firmness of the clot (shear elastic modulus strength, SEMS; in units of dyn/cm^2). G is determined from the log-derivative of MA.

Coagulation Index (CI): mathematically combines R-time, K-time, α-angle, and MA into a single relative expression of coagulability (normal. −3.0 to 3.0). A CI >3.0 indicates the sample is hypercoagulable; a CI <−3.0 indicates that the sample is hypocoagulable.

---

by stimulation of a whole-blood sample with kaolin alone may have higher sensitivity in detection of low levels of fibrinolysis.[105]

Goal-directed DCR has been shown to significantly improve outcomes by reducing bleeding and diminishing transfusion requirements.[106] Specific and rapid correction of coagulopathies is more effective, which improves outcomes due to attenuation of an autoinflammatory response.[107] Consistent with management of hemorrhage in trauma patients, implementation of POC viscoelastography-based protocols for the management of hemorrhage in cardiovascular surgical patients has been shown to reduce perioperative transfusion requirements, along with transfusion-related adverse events. This includes a decrease in thromboembolic complications and an improved 6-month survival rate.[108]

Pharmacologic Adjuncts

Several studies suggest that the risk of death after trauma correlates with the degree of fibrinolysis present in trauma patients on admission to the hospital, whereas the presence of hyperfibrinolysis in patients with severe injuries, many requiring DCR, is associated with an extraordinarily high mortality.[109] Moreover, CRASH-2, an unusually large, multinational, randomized controlled trial, which has been highly publicized, reported a reduction in mortality (albeit small) in trauma patients treated within 3 hours of injury with an antifibrinolytic agent, tranexamic acid (TXA).[110] CRASH-2 is not without considerable controversy, however, including a finding reported in CRASH-2 that treatment with TXA after 3 hours of injury is associated with an increase in mortality.[111] In addition, recent data indicate that many injured patients may be at increased risk for complications or death due to down-regulation of fibrinolysis, suggesting that the routine use of TXA in trauma patients may be contraindicated.[59]

Fibrinogen concentrate given during resuscitation correlates with significant improvement in coagulation parameters, and substantially reduces requirements for RBC, fresh frozen plasma, and platelet transfusions. In Europe, fibrinogen concentrate is now used in place of allogeneic blood products as a first-line treatment of hypofibrinogemia, including acquired hypofibrinogenemia developing in the trauma patient.[112] Fibrinogen concentrate is commercially available in the United States and approved by the Food and Drug Administration (FDA) to treat hereditary fibrinogen disorders. Fibrinogen concentrate to correct acquired fibrinogen deficiency complicating HS, however, has not yet been approved by the FDA.[113]

Activated recombinant human FVII (rhVIIa) has a limited role in DCR but may be useful in unusual circumstances. As an example, acquired FVIII deficiency of variable degrees develops in association with pregnancy approximately 8% to 15% of the time, which resolves within 30 months of delivery.[114] Hemostatic resuscitation for hemorrhage in a pregnant patient with FVIII deficiency may require rhVIIa in addition to specific blood components to manage disruption of the hemostatic mechanism.

Homeostatic Resuscitation

Acidosis

There are multiple adverse systemic responses to acidosis (pH $\leq$7.20).[115] These include decreased cardiac contractility and dysrhythmias. Cardiogenic shock contributes significantly to hypoperfusion by abolishing an important mechanism of compensation for hypovolemia in the exsanguinating patient. Acidosis desensitizes peripheral vasculature adrenergic receptors to endogenous catecholamines,[116] which disables other compensatory mechanisms that are active in response to HS, including the activation of inflammation and the suppression of immunity.[117] Acidosis also inhibits platelet activation, diminishes coagulation factor activity, and accelerates breakdown of fibrinogen.[118] The presence of excess H^+ destabilizes crucial interactions between phospholipid platforms in activated platelets and coagulation

factor complexes, further diminishing coagulation potential in the patient in HS.[119] Thus increases in base deficit lead to an increase in the mortality of the hemorrhaging patient.[120] The detrimental effects of acidosis and coagulopathy are compounded when associated with hypothermia (core temperature <34°C), which is underscored by the phrase, "lethal triad of trauma."

Administration of tris(hydroxymethyl)-aminomethane (THAM) is more effective than bicarbonate at correcting the deep acid-base imbalance of lactic acidosis due to HS.[121] The initial loading dose of a 0.3 mol/L-solution of THAM acetate is equal to lean body weight (kg) $\times$ base deficit (mmol/L), and the maximum dose for a 24-hour period is 15 mmol/kg, or 3.5 L for a 70-kg patient.[121] THAM does not lower intracellular pH, reduce serum ionized calcium, or affect serum osmolality.[117] Treating acidosis with THAM leads to a distortion in the anion gap, decreasing the usefulness of this number in the determination of different treatment strategies during DCR.

Hypothermia

A decrease in core body temperature negatively affects the enzymatic specificity constants of coagulation factors in the hemostatic pathway and increases mortality of patients in HS. For each 1°C drop in temperature, coagulation factor activity is reduced by approximately 10% to 15%. This is exacerbated by factor depletion secondary to dilution or consumption.[122] Hypothermia has multiple effects on coagulation including the inhibition of endogenous anticoagulants as well as coagulation factor activity. A more important clinical effect of hypothermia on coagulation is inhibition of von Willebrand factor–platelet glycoprotein Ib-IX-V interactions,[123] which mediate platelet adherence in high-flow conditions. TEG or ROTEM can be performed at a patient's actual core temperature. Standard assays are performed after serum has been warmed to 37°C. TEG for example, may reveal a prolonged R-time (enzymatic reaction time), lower K-time (rate of clot formation), and lower α-angle (clot formation time).[124] Hypothermic-mediated inhibition of clotting times and clotting rates synergize with hemorrhage-mediated reduction in clot strength (maximum amplitude [MA] by TEG determination), which explains in part the significant worsening of hemorrhage-associated coagulopathy caused by reduced core body temperature.[125] Although mild hypothermia may increase cardiac output, moderate or severe hypothermia can depress myocardial contractility and reduce cardiac output.[126] The reduction in cardiac output in a hypothermic patient is exacerbated by atrial and/or ventricular tachyarrhythmias.[127]

Hypothermia is induced or perpetuated by infusion of room-temperature fluids or cold blood products. In a hemorrhaging patient, metabolism is significantly diminished, and consequently heat production is reduced.[128] External rewarming methods help to prevent heat loss but transfer virtually no heat to the patient.

Divalent cation deficiency

Reduced circulating levels of calcium and magnesium are the most common adverse homeostatic events in DCR and are due to citrate toxicity. Blood is stored in citrate, a calcium binding agent, and therefore large amounts of citrate accompany blood components transfused in massive amounts. One unit of RBCs contains 3 g of citrate, which can be metabolized by a normal liver within 5 minutes. Transfusion rates higher than 1 unit every 5 minutes, often the case in DCR, lead to citrate accumulation and hypocalcemia. Diminished citrate clearance due to preexisting liver disease, or impaired hepatic function secondary to hypothermia, shock liver, or high grades of liver injury, potentiate the development of citrate toxicity and hypocalcemia.[129] Hypocalcemia reduces myocardial contractility and impairs maintenance of vasomotor tone. Hypomagnesemia and hypocalcemia are associated with disruption of myocardial repolarization. This is characterized by a prolongation of the QT interval and places the patient at a risk for development of torsades de pointes.[130]

To prevent hypocalcemia during DCR, 1 to 2 ampules of calcium gluconate or calcium chloride may be administered intravenously at the onset of DCR and then after every 4 to 8 U of RBCs or plasma that are transfused. A 10-mL ampule of calcium chloride contains 270 mg of calcium. Magnesium for intravenous injection is supplied as magnesium sulfate in 50% and 12.5% solutions. A solution of 6 g of magnesium sulfate (48 mEq) in 250 mL of saline is infused over 3 hours for serum magnesium less than 1 mEq/L.

Hypoxia

The improved early survival of DCR strategies associated with high plasma:RBC ratios may be nullified by an increase in late hospital mortality secondary to multisystem organ failure.[131] TRALI is the leading cause of mortality that develops during or within 6 hours after the transfusion of 1 or more units of blood or blood components, including platelets.[132] TRALI represents approximately 38% of confirmed transfusion-related fatalities reported to the FDA in the past 5 years.[133]

Transfusion-associated circulatory overload (TACO) during DCR is caused by the infusion of blood products at a high rate, in large volumes, or both. Signs and symptoms of TACO include acute onset of hypoxia, tachypnea, tachycardia, and rapidly falling oxygen saturation as measured by pulse oximetry (SpO_2).[134] TACO is associated, predictably, with a previous medical history of congestive heart failure, coronary artery disease, previous coronary bypass surgery, and atrial fibrillation.[135] TRALI and TACO are managed with low tidal volume mechanical ventilation set to reduce pressures sufficiently to minimize atelectrauma, yet maintain recruitment of alveoli.

Minimizing ischemia-reperfusion injury

Reperfusion injury is caused by a rapid restoration of normal blood flow to hypoperfused tissue during DCR. Reperfusion induces nonspecific activation of coagulation/fibrinolysis system as well as activation of innate immune processes. This occurs in concert with the down-regulation of endogenous anticoagulants and anti-inflammatory pathways.[136,137] The dissemination of constitutive intracellular molecules released from disrupted cells in areas of ischemia and damaged tissue underlies, in part, the pathophysiology of reperfusion injury. These molecules contain a so-called damage-associated molecular pattern (DAMP) motif as part of the molecular structure. DAMPs are recognized by pattern recognition receptors (PRRs). Binding of DAMP ligands to PRRs mediates activation of many host innate immune systems. This creates the potential for systemic autoinflammatory tissue damage and organ failure.[138] Circulating levels of high mobility group box 1 protein (HMGB1), the prototype host molecule bearing a DAMP motif, are increased during HS. HMGB1 binds to a PRR, Toll-like receptor 4 (TLR4) expressed on several cell types, such as dendritic cells, neutrophils, macrophages, lymphocytes, endothelial cells, and platelets. HMGB1-TLR4 interactions activate proinflammatory activities,[139,140] which mediate an autoinflammatory response expressed clinically as a systemic inflammatory response syndrome.[141,142] RBCs stored for long periods release free hemoglobin containing DAMP structures, which may contribute in unexpected ways to the adverse effects of MT.

Diffuse interstitial edema and cellular swelling are the consequences of systemic autoinflammatory syndrome. Marked splanchnic hypoperfusion is a characteristic feature of the compensatory mechanisms that operate in response to massive blood loss. Subsequent reperfusion of hypoperfused gut mucosa during

DCR produces significant bowel wall edema leading to intra-abdominal hypertension (IAH).[143,144] Bowel edema during reperfusion occurs early, and IAH may progress to intra-abdominal compartment syndrome, which is associated with organ failure.[145] IAH produces a reduction in inferior vena cava blood flow leading to a reduction in right ventricular (RV) preload.[146,147] RV dilatation may develop as a response to increased RV afterload, causing a decrease in ejection fraction. RV dilatation impinges on the ventricular septum, which, due to ventricular interdependence, decreases left ventricular preload. This leads to a further reduction in cardiac output.[148]

SUMMARY

Catastrophic hemorrhage from severe facial trauma or as a complication of complex oral and maxillofacial surgery requires immediate and massive resuscitation to simultaneously correct several hemodynamic, hemostatic, and homeostatic disorders. Resuscitation of this magnitude requires critical decisions that often must be reached with little time and without sufficient clinical data about patients on which to base initiation of such a crucial, potentially dangerous, and resource-intensive treatment. Against this foreboding backdrop, the development of comprehensive DCR protocols used currently in many trauma centers has led to a substantial improvement in the survival for patients in profound HS. Prior to 1990, the survival rate of patients with acute severe blood loss ranged from 10% to 40%. With recent progress in resuscitation practices, including a better understanding of the complex physiology of HS, recognition and management of TAC, and attention to the profound disruption in homeostasis that complicates the resuscitation of hemorrhaging patients, current survival rates have improved considerably.[149] Recent advances in DCR are based on results from sophisticated laboratory and clinical investigations. Consequently, the management of exsanguinating patients requires surgeons across several specialties to now possess a basic familiarity with multiple clinical and scientific disciplines.

REFERENCES

1. Schochl H, Grassetto A, Schlimp CJ. Management of hemorrhage in trauma. J Cardiothorac Vasc Anesth 2013;27:S35–43.
2. Weiskopf RB, Ness PM. Transfusion for remote damage control resuscitation. Transfusion 2013; 53(Suppl 1):1S–5S.
3. Ball CG. Damage control resuscitation: history, theory and technique. Can J Surg 2014;57:55–60.
4. Gonzalez E, Moore EE, Moore HB, et al. Trauma-induced coagulopathy: an institution's 35 year perspective on practice and research. Scand J Surg 2014;103:89–103.
5. Jenkins DH, Rappold JF, Badloe JF, et al. Trauma hemostasis and oxygenation research position paper on remote damage control resuscitation: definitions, current practice, and knowledge gaps. Shock 2014;41(Suppl 1):3–12.
6. Johansson PI, Stensballe J, Oliveri R, et al. How I treat patients with massive hemorrhage. Blood 2014;124(20):3052–8.
7. Pohlman TH, Walsh M, Aversa J, et al. Damage control resuscitation. Blood Rev 2015;29:251–62.
8. Cotton BA, Au BK, Nunez TC, et al. Predefined massive transfusion protocols are associated with a reduction in organ failure and postinjury complications. J Trauma 2009;66:41–8.
9. Cotton BA, Reddy N, Hatch QM, et al. Damage control resuscitation is associated with a reduction in resuscitation volumes and improvement in survival in 390 damage control laparotomy patients. Ann Surg 2011;254:598–605.
10. Roback JD, Caldwell S, Carson J, et al, American Association for the Study of Liver, American Academy of Pediatrics, United States Army, American Society of Anesthesiology; American Society of Hematology. Evidence-based practice guidelines for plasma transfusion. Transfusion 2010;50: 1227–39.
11. Cryer HG, Nathens AB, Bulger EM, et al. ACS TQIP massive transfusion in trauma guidelines. ACS Trauma Quality Improvement Program, vol. 2015. Chicago, Il: American College of Surgeons Committee on Trauma; 2013.
12. Wiegmann TL, Mintz PD. The growing role of AABB clinical practice guidelines in improving patient care. Transfusion 2015;55:935–6.
13. Mutschler M, Nienaber U, Brockamp T, et al, TraumaRegister DGU. Renaissance of base deficit for the initial assessment of trauma patients: a base deficit-based classification for hypovolemic shock developed on data from 16,305 patients derived from the TraumaRegister DGU(R). Crit Care 2013; 17:R42.
14. Shere-Wolfe RF, Galvagno SM Jr, Grissom TE. Critical care considerations in the management of the trauma patient following initial resuscitation. Scand J Trauma Resusc Emerg Med 2012;20:68.
15. Gann DS, Drucker WR. Hemorrhagic shock. J Trauma Acute Care Surg 2013;75:888–95.
16. Orlinsky M, Shoemaker W, Reis ED, et al. Current controversies in shock and resuscitation. Surg Clin North Am 2001;81:1217–62.

17. Guan J, Jin DD, Jin LJ, et al. Apoptosis in organs of rats in early stage after polytrauma combined with shock. J Trauma 2002;52:104–11.

18. Cowley RA, Mergner WJ, Fisher RS, et al. The subcellular pathology of shock in trauma patients: studies using the immediate autopsy. Am Surg 1979;45:255–69.

19. Dunser MW, Takala J, Brunauer A, et al. Re-thinking resuscitation: leaving blood pressure cosmetics behind and moving forward to permissive hypotension and a tissue perfusion-based approach. Crit Care 2013;17:326.

20. Guly HR, Bouamra O, Spiers M, et al. Vital signs and estimated blood loss in patients with major trauma: testing the validity of the ATLS classification of hypovolaemic shock. Resuscitation 2011; 82:556–9.

21. Strehlow MC. Early identification of shock in critically ill patients. Emerg Med Clin North Am 2010; 28:57–66.

22. Vandromme MJ, Griffin RL, Weinberg JA, et al. Lactate is a better predictor than systolic blood pressure for determining blood requirement and mortality: could prehospital measures improve trauma triage? J Am Coll Surg 2010;210:861–7, 867–9.

23. Wilson M, Davis DP, Coimbra R. Diagnosis and monitoring of hemorrhagic shock during the initial resuscitation of multiple trauma patients: a review. J Emerg Med 2003;24:413–22.

24. Brasel KJ, Guse C, Gentilello LM, et al. Heart rate: is it truly a vital sign? J Trauma 2007;62:812–7.

25. Cannon CM, Braxton CC, Kling-Smith M, et al. Utility of the shock index in predicting mortality in traumatically injured patients. J Trauma 2009;67:1426–30.

26. Little RA, Kirkman E, Driscoll P, et al. Preventable deaths after injury: why are the traditional 'vital' signs poor indicators of blood loss? J Accid Emerg Med 1995;12:1–14.

27. Vandromme MJ, Griffin RL, Kerby JD, et al. Identifying risk for massive transfusion in the relatively normotensive patient: utility of the prehospital shock index. J Trauma 2011;70:384–8.

28. Zarzaur BL, Croce MA, Fischer PE, et al. New vitals after injury: shock index for the young and age x shock index for the old. J Surg Res 2008;147: 229–36.

29. Zarzaur BL, Croce MA, Magnotti LJ, et al. Identifying life-threatening shock in the older injured patient: an analysis of the National Trauma Data Bank. J Trauma 2010;68:1134–8.

30. Mitra B, Fitzgerald M, Chan J. The utility of a shock index >/= 1 as an indication for pre-hospital oxygen carrier administration in major trauma. Injury 2014;45:61–5.

31. Ardagh MW, Hodgson T, Shaw L, et al. Pulse rate over pressure evaluation (ROPE) is useful in the assessment of compensated haemorrhagic shock. Emerg Med (Fremantle) 2001;13:43–6.

32. Campbell R, Ardagh MW, Than M. Validation of the pulse rate over pressure evaluation index as a detector of early occult hemorrhage: a prospective observational study. J Trauma Acute Care Surg 2012;73:286–8.

33. Juern J, Khatri V, Weigelt J. Base excess: a review. J Trauma Acute Care Surg 2012;73:27–32.

34. Dunham CM, Watson LA, Cooper C. Base deficit level indicating major injury is increased with ethanol. J Emerg Med 2000;18:165–71.

35. Cardenas JC, Wade CE, Holcomb JB. Mechanisms of trauma-induced coagulopathy. Curr Opin Hematol 2014;21:404–9.

36. Davenport RA, Brohi K. Cause of trauma-induced coagulopathy. Curr Opin Anaesthesiol 2016;29: 212–9.

37. Noel P, Cashen S, Patel B. Trauma-Induced Coagulopathy: From Biology to Therapy. Semin Hematol 2013;50:259–69.

38. MacLeod JB, Lynn M, McKenney MG, et al. Early coagulopathy predicts mortality in trauma. J Trauma 2003;55:39–44.

39. Brohi K, Cohen MJ, Ganter MT, et al. Acute coagulopathy of trauma: hypoperfusion induces systemic anticoagulation and hyperfibrinolysis. J Trauma 2008;64:1211–7.

40. Cohen MJ, Kutcher M, Redick B, et al. Clinical and mechanistic drivers of acute traumatic coagulopathy. J Trauma Acute Care Surg 2013;75:S40–7.

41. Haywood-Watson RJ, Holcomb JB, Gonzalez EA, et al. Modulation of syndecan-1 shedding after hemorrhagic shock and resuscitation. PLoS One 2011;6:e23530.

42. Johansson PI, SØRensen AM, Perner A, et al. High sCD40L levels early after trauma are associated with enhanced shock, sympathoadrenal activation, tissue and endothelial damage, coagulopathy and mortality. J Thromb Haemost 2012;10:207–16.

43. Johansson PI, Stensballe J, Rasmussen LS, et al. High circulating adrenaline levels at admission predict increased mortality after trauma. J Trauma Acute Care Surg 2012;72:428–36.

44. Mann KG, Freeman K. TACTIC: Trans-Agency Consortium for Trauma-Induced Coagulopathy. J Thromb Haemost 2015;13(Suppl 1):S63–71.

45. Martin FA, Murphy RP, Cummins PM. Thrombomodulin and the vascular endothelium: insights into functional, regulatory, and therapeutic aspects. Am J Physiol Heart Circ Physiol 2013;304:H1585–97.

46. Gando S, Otomo Y. Local hemostasis, immunothrombosis, and systemic disseminated intravascular coagulation in trauma and traumatic shock. Crit Care 2015;19:72.

47. Becker BF, Chappell D, Bruegger D, et al. Therapeutic strategies targeting the endothelial

glycocalyx: acute deficits, but great potential. Cardiovasc Res 2010;87:300–10.

48. Ostrowski SR, Johansson PI. Endothelial glycocalyx degradation induces endogenous heparinization in patients with severe injury and early traumatic coagulopathy. J Trauma Acute Care Surg 2012;73:60–6.

49. Castellino FJ, Chapman MP, Donahue DL, et al. Traumatic brain injury causes platelet adenosine diphosphate and arachidonic acid receptor inhibition independent of hemorrhagic shock in humans and rats. J Trauma Acute Care Surg 2014;76:1169–76.

50. Ramsey MT, Fabian TC, Shahan CP, et al. A prospective study of platelet function in trauma patients. J Trauma Acute Care Surg 2016;80(5): 726–33.

51. Johansson PI, Sorensen AM, Perner A, et al. Disseminated intravascular coagulation or acute coagulopathy of trauma shock early after trauma? An observational study. Crit Care 2011;15:R272.

52. Gando S, Wada H, Kim HK, et al. Scientific, Standardization Committee on DICotI. Comparison of disseminated intravascular coagulation in trauma with coagulopathy of trauma/acute coagulopathy of trauma-shock. J Thromb Haemost 2012;10: 2593–5.

53. Schochl H, Voelckel W, Maegele M, et al. Trauma-associated hyperfibrinolysis. Hamostaseologie 2012;32:22–7.

54. Okafor ON, Gorog DA. Endogenous fibrinolysis: an important mediator of thrombus formation and cardiovascular risk. J Am Coll Cardiol 2015;65: 1683–99.

55. Schuster V, Hugle B, Tefs K. Plasminogen deficiency. J Thromb Haemost 2007;5:2315–22.

56. Mehta R, Shapiro AD. Plasminogen deficiency. Haemophilia 2008;14:1261–8.

57. Raza I, Davenport R, Rourke C, et al. The incidence and magnitude of fibrinolytic activation in trauma patients. J Thromb Haemost 2013;11:307–14.

58. Bolliger D, Szlam F, Levy JH, et al. Haemodilution-induced profibrinolytic state is mitigated by fresh-frozen plasma: implications for early haemostatic intervention in massive haemorrhage. Br J Anaesth 2010;104:318–25.

59. Moore EE, Moore HB, Gonzalez E, et al. Postinjury fibrinolysis shutdown: Rationale for selective tranexamic acid. J Trauma Acute Care Surg 2015; 78:S65–9.

60. Chapman MP, Moore EE, Moore HB, et al. The "Black Diamond": rapid thrombelastography identifies lethal hyperfibrinolysis. J Trauma Acute Care Surg 2015;79(6):925–9.

61. Hunt BJ, Segal H. Hyperfibrinolysis. J Clin Pathol 1996;49:958.

62. Stachurska J, Latallo Z, Kopec M. Inhibition of platelet aggregation by dialysable fibrinogen

degradation products (FDP). Thromb Diath Haemorrh 1970;23:91–8.

63. vanDeWater L, Carr JM, Aronson D, et al. Analysis of elevated fibrin(ogen) degradation product levels in patients with liver disease. Blood 1986; 67:1468–73.

64. Khan S, Allard S, Weaver A, et al. A major haemorrhage protocol improves the delivery of blood component therapy and reduces waste in trauma massive transfusion. Injury 2013;44:587–92.

65. Holcomb JB, Gumbert S. Potential value of protocols in substantially bleeding trauma patients. Curr Opin Anaesthesiol 2013;26:215–20.

66. Lubarsky DA, Smith LR, Sladen RN, et al. Defining the relationship of oxygen delivery and consumption: use of biologic system models. J Surg Res 1995;58:503–8.

67. Omert LA, Billiar TR. Hemorrhagic shock: from physiology to molecular biology. In: Pinski M, editor. Applied cardiovascular physiology, Vol 28: Berlin: Springer; 1997. p. 209–16.

68. D'Alessandro A, Kriebardis AG, Rinalducci S, et al. An update on red blood cell storage lesions, as gleaned through biochemistry and omics technologies. Transfusion 2015;55:205–19.

69. Zubair AC. Clinical impact of blood storage lesions. Am J Hematol 2010;85:117–22.

70. Kim-Shapiro DB, Lee J, Gladwin MT. Storage lesion: role of red blood cell breakdown. Transfusion 2011;51:844–51.

71. Tinmouth A, Fergusson D, Yee IC, et al, Canadian Critical Care Trials Group. Clinical consequences of red cell storage in the critically ill. Transfusion 2006;46:2014–27.

72. Almac E, Bezemer R, Hilarius-Stokman PM, et al. Red blood cell storage increases hypoxia-induced nitric oxide bioavailability and methemoglobin formation in vitro and in vivo. Transfusion 2014;54:3178–85.

73. Young JA, Lichtman MA, Cohen J. Reduced red cell 2,3-diphosphoglycerate and adenosine triphosphate, hypophosphatemia, and increased hemoglobin-oxygen affinity after cardiac surgery. Circulation 1973;47:1313–8.

74. Watkins GM, Rabelo A, Pizak LF, et al. The left shifted oxyhemoglobin curve in sepsis: a preventable defect. Ann Surg 1974;180:213–20.

75. Raat NJH, Ince C. Oxygenating the microcirculation: the perspective from blood transfusion and blood storage. Vox Sang 2007;93:12–8.

76. Middelburg RA, Borkent B, Jansen M, et al. Storage time of blood products and transfusion-related acute lung injury. Transfusion 2012;52:658–67.

77. Hampton DA, Wiles C, Fabricant LJ, et al. Cryopreserved red blood cells are superior to standard liquid red blood cells. J Trauma Acute Care Surg 2014;77:20–7.

78. Johansson PI, Hansen MB, Sorensen H. Transfusion practice in massively bleeding patients: time for a change? Vox Sang 2005;89:92–6.

79. Cushing M, Shaz BH. Blood transfusion in trauma patients: unresolved questions. Minerva Anestesiol 2011;77:349–59.

80. Gutierrez MC, Goodnough LT, Druzin M, et al. Postpartum hemorrhage treated with a massive transfusion protocol at a tertiary obstetric center: a retrospective study. Int J Obstet Anesth 2012;21:230–5.

81. Holcomb JB, Pati S. Optimal trauma resuscitation with plasma as the primary resuscitative fluid: the surgeon's perspective. Hematology Am Soc Hematol Educ Program 2013;2013:656–9.

82. Holcomb JB, Wade CE, Michalek JE, et al. Increased plasma and platelet to red blood cell ratios improves outcome in 466 massively transfused civilian trauma patients. Ann Surg 2008;248:447–58.

83. Johansson PI, Stensballe J. Effect of Haemostatic Control Resuscitation on mortality in massively bleeding patients: a before and after study. Vox Sang 2009;96:111–8.

84. Johansson PI, Stensballe J, Ostrowski SR. Current management of massive hemorrhage in trauma. Scand J Trauma Resusc Emerg Med 2012;20:47.

85. Riskin DJ, Tsai TC, Riskin L, et al. Massive transfusion protocols: the role of aggressive resuscitation versus product ratio in mortality reduction. J Am Coll Surg 2009;209:198–205.

86. Holcomb JB. Optimal use of blood products in severely injured trauma patients. Hematology Am Soc Hematol Educ Program 2010;2010:465–9.

87. Holcomb JB, Tilley BC, Baraniuk S, et al. Transfusion of plasma, platelets, and red blood cells in a 1:1:1 vs a 1:1:2 ratio and mortality in patients with severe trauma: the PROPPR randomized clinical trial. JAMA 2015;313:471–82.

88. Hess JR, Holcomb JB. Resuscitating PROPPRly. Transfusion 2015;55(6):1362–4.

89. Buchta C, Felfernig M, Hocker P, et al. Stability of coagulation factors in thawed, solvent/detergent-treated plasma during storage at 4 degrees C for 6 days. Vox Sang 2004;87:182–6.

90. Chhibber V, Greene M, Vauthrin M, et al. Is group A thawed plasma suitable as the first option for emergency release transfusion? (CME). Transfusion 2014;54:1751–5.

91. Cooling L. Going from A to B: the safety of incompatible group A plasma for emergency release in trauma and massive transfusion patients. Transfusion 2014;54:1695–7.

92. Mehr CR, Gupta R, von Recklinghausen FM, et al. Balancing risk and benefit: maintenance of a thawed Group A plasma inventory for trauma patients requiring massive transfusion. J Trauma Acute Care Surg 2013;74:1425–31.

93. Zielinski MD, Johnson PM, Jenkins D, et al. Emergency use of prethawed Group A plasma in trauma patients. J Trauma Acute Care Surg 2013;74:69–74.

94. Levy JH, Szlam F, Tanaka KA, et al. Fibrinogen and hemostasis: a primary hemostatic target for the management of acquired bleeding. Anesth Analg 2012;114:261–74.

95. Meyer MA, Ostrowski SR, Sorensen AM, et al. Fibrinogen in trauma, an evaluation of thrombelastography and rotational thromboelastometry fibrinogen assays. J Surg Res 2015;194:581–90.

96. Rourke C, Curry N, Khan S, et al. Fibrinogen levels during trauma hemorrhage, response to replacement therapy, and association with patient outcomes. J Thromb Haemost 2012;10:1342–51.

97. Kushimoto S, Shibata Y, Yamamoto Y. Implications of fibrinogenolysis in patients with closed head injury. J Neurotrauma 2003;20:357–63.

98. Martini WZ, Holcomb JB. Acidosis and coagulopathy: the differential effects on fibrinogen synthesis and breakdown in pigs. Ann Surg 2007;246:831–5.

99. Johansson PI. Coagulation monitoring of the bleeding traumatized patient. Curr Opin Anaesthesiol 2012;25:235–41.

100. Bolliger D, Seeberger MD, Tanaka KA. Principles and practice of thromboelastography in clinical coagulation management and transfusion practice. Transfus Med Rev 2012;26:1–13.

101. Rumph B, Bolliger D, Narang N, et al. In vitro comparative study of hemostatic components in warfarin-treated and fibrinogen-deficient plasma. J Cardiothorac Vasc Anesth 2010;24:408–12.

102. Johansson PI. Goal-directed hemostatic resuscitation for massively bleeding patients: the Copenhagen concept. Transfus Apher Sci 2010;43:401–5.

103. da Luz LT, Nascimento B, Rizoli S. Thrombelastography (TEG(R)): practical considerations on its clinical use in trauma resuscitation. Scand J Trauma Resusc Emerg Med 2013;21:29.

104. Jeger V, Zimmermann H, Exadaktylos AK. Can RapidTEG accelerate the search for coagulopathies in the patient with multiple injuries? J Trauma 2009;66:1253–7.

105. Genet GF, Ostrowski SR, Sorensen AM, et al. Detection of tPA-induced hyperfibrinolysis in whole blood by RapidTEG, KaolinTEG, and functional fibrinogenTEG in healthy individuals. Clin Appl Thromb Hemost 2012;18:638–44.

106. Kashuk JL, Moore EE, Wohlauer M, et al. Initial experiences with point-of-care rapid thrombelastography for management of life-threatening postinjury coagulopathy. Transfusion 2012;52:23–33.

107. Kashuk JL, Moore EE, Sawyer M, et al. Postinjury coagulopathy management: goal directed resuscitation via POC thrombelastography. Ann Surg 2010;251:604–14.

108. Gorlinger K, Dirkmann D, Hanke AA. Potential value of transfusion protocols in cardiac surgery. Curr Opin Anaesthesiol 2013;26:230–43.

109. Napolitano LM, Cohen MJ, Cotton BA, et al. Tranexamic acid in trauma: how should we use it? J Trauma Acute Care Surg 2013;74:1575–86.

110. Shakur H, Roberts I, Bautista R, et al. Effects of tranexamic acid on death, vascular occlusive events, and blood transfusion in trauma patients with significant haemorrhage (CRASH-2): a randomised, placebo-controlled trial. Lancet 2010; 376:23–32.

111. Binz S, McCollester J, Thomas S, et al. CRASH-2 study of tranexamic acid to treat bleeding in trauma patients: a controversy fueled by science and social media. J Blood Transfus 2015;2015: 874920.

112. Schochl H, Nienaber U, Maegele M, et al. Transfusion in trauma: thromboelastometry-guided coagulation factor concentrate-based therapy versus standard fresh frozen plasma-based therapy. Crit Care 2011;15:R83.

113. Harr JN, Moore EE, Ghasabyan A, et al. Functional fibrinogen assay indicates that fibrinogen is critical in correcting abnormal clot strength following trauma. Shock 2013;39:45–9.

114. Bonfanti C, Crestani S, Frattini F, et al. Role of rituximab in the treatment of postpartum acquired haemophilia A: a systematic review of the literature. Blood Transfus 2015;13:396–400.

115. Schotola H, Sossalla S, Rajab TK, et al. Influence of mild metabolic acidosis on cardiac contractility and isoprenaline response in isolated ovine myocardium. Artif Organs 2011;35:1065–74.

116. Kraut JA, Madias NE. Metabolic acidosis: pathophysiology, diagnosis and management. Nat Rev Nephrol 2010;6:274–85.

117. Kraut JA, Madias NE. Treatment of acute metabolic acidosis: a pathophysiologic approach. Nat Rev Nephrol 2012;8:589–601.

118. Martini WZ. Coagulopathy by hypothermia and acidosis: mechanisms of thrombin generation and fibrinogen availability. J Trauma 2009;67:202–8.

119. Murthi SB, Stansbury LG, Dutton RP, et al. Transfusion medicine in trauma patients: an update. Expert Rev Hematol 2011;4:527–37.

120. Tremblay LN, Feliciano DV, Rozycki GS. Assessment of initial base deficit as a predictor of outcome: mechanism of injury does make a difference. Am Surg 2002;68:689–93.

121. Nahas GG, Sutin KM, Fermon C, et al. Guidelines for the treatment of acidaemia with THAM. Drugs 1998;55:191–224.

122. Wolberg AS, Meng ZH, Monroe DM 3rd, et al. A systematic evaluation of the effect of temperature on coagulation enzyme activity and platelet function. J Trauma 2004;56:1221–8.

123. Kermode JC, Zheng Q, Milner EP. Marked temperature dependence of the platelet calcium signal induced by human von Willebrand factor. Blood 1999;94:199–207.

124. Douning LK, Ramsay MA, Swygert TH, et al. Temperature corrected thrombelastography in hypothermic patients. Anesth Analg 1995;81:608–11.

125. Martini WZ, Cortez DS, Dubick MA, et al. Thrombelastography is better than PT, aPTT, and activated clotting time in detecting clinically relevant clotting abnormalities after hypothermia, hemorrhagic shock and resuscitation in pigs. J Trauma 2008; 65:535–43.

126. Peng RY, Bongard FS. Hypothermia in trauma patients. J Am Coll Surg 1999;188:685–96.

127. Okada M. The cardiac rhythm in accidental hypothermia. J Electrocardiol 1984;17:123–8.

128. Gentilello LM, Moujaes S. Treatment of hypothermia in trauma victims: thermodynamic considerations. J Intensive Care Med 1995;10:5–14.

129. Sihler KC, Napolitano LM. Complications of massive transfusion. Chest 2010;137:209–20.

130. Passman R, Kadish A. Polymorphic ventricular tachycardia, long Q-T syndrome, and torsades de pointes. Med Clin North Am 2001;85:321–41.

131. Moore FA, Moore EE, Sauaia A. Blood transfusion. An independent risk factor for postinjury multiple organ failure. Arch Surg 1997;132:620–4.

132. Toy P, Gajic O, Bacchetti P, et al, TRALI Study Group. Transfusion-related acute lung injury: incidence and risk factors. Blood 2012;119:1757–67.

133. FDA Center for Biologics Evaluation and Research. Fatalities reported to the FDA following blood collection and transfusion. Annual Summary for Fiscal Year 2014. Available at: http://www.fda. gov/downloads/BiologicsBloodVaccines/Safety Availability/ReportaProblem/TransfusionDonation Fatalities/UCM459461.pdf. Accessed July 18, 2016.

134. Palfi M, Berg S, Ernerudh J, et al. A randomized controlled trial oftransfusion-related acute lung injury: is plasma from multiparous blood donors dangerous? Transfusion 2001;41:317–22.

135. Murphy EL, Kwaan N, Looney MR, et al. Risk factors and outcomes in transfusion-associated circulatory overload. Am J Med 2013;126(357):e29–38.

136. Conway EM. Thrombomodulin and its role in inflammation. Semin Immunopathol 2012;34:107–25.

137. Niesler U, Palmer A, Froba JS, et al. Role of alveolar macrophages in the regulation of local and systemic inflammation after lung contusion. J Trauma Acute Care Surg 2014;76:386–93.

138. Neal MD, Raval JS, Triulzi DJ, et al. Innate immune activation after transfusion of stored red blood cells. Transfus Med Rev 2013;27:113–8.

139. Bae JS, Rezaie AR. Activated protein C inhibits high mobility group box 1 signaling in endothelial cells. Blood 2011;118:3952–9.

140. Treutiger CJ, Mullins GE, Johansson AS, et al. High mobility group 1 B-box mediates activation of human endothelium. J Intern Med 2003;254:375–85.

141. McGhan LJ, Jaroszewski DE. The role of toll-like receptor-4 in the development of multi-organ failure following traumatic haemorrhagic shock and resuscitation. Injury 2012;43:129–36.

142. Prince JM, Levy RM, Yang R, et al. Toll-like receptor-4 signaling mediates hepatic injury and systemic inflammation in hemorrhagic shock. J Am Coll Surg 2006;202:407–17.

143. Cheatham ML, Malbrain ML. Cardiovascular implications of abdominal compartment syndrome. Acta Clin Belg 2007;62(Suppl 1):98–112.

144. Fabian TC. Damage control in trauma: laparotomy wound management acute to chronic. Surg Clin North Am 2007;87:73–93.

145. Cheatham ML. Abdominal compartment syndrome. Curr Opin Crit Care 2009;15:154–62.

146. Barnes GE, Laine GA, Giam PY, et al. Cardiovascular responses to elevation of intra-abdominal hydrostatic pressure. Am J Physiol 1985;248: R208–13.

147. Cullen DJ, Coyle JP, Teplick R, et al. Cardiovascular, pulmonary, and renal effects of massively increased intra-abdominal pressure in critically ill patients. Crit Care Med 1989;17:118–21.

148. Cheatham ML, Nelson LD, Chang MC, et al. Right ventricular end-diastolic volume index as a predictor of preload status in patients on positive end-expiratory pressure. Crit Care Med 1998;26: 1801–6.

149. Kobayashi L, Costantini TW, Coimbra R. Hypovolemic shock resuscitation. Surg Clin North Am 2012; 92:1403–23.

Index

Oral Maxillofacial Surg Clin N Am 28 (2016) 569–575

http://dx.doi.org/10.1016/S1042-3699(16)30085-1

1042-3699/16/$ – see front matter

Moving?

Make sure your subscription moves with you!

To notify us of your new address, find your **Clinics Account Number** (located on your mailing label above your name), and contact customer service at:

Email: journalscustomerservice-usa@elsevier.com

800-654-2452 (subscribers in the U.S. & Canada)
314-447-8871 (subscribers outside of the U.S. & Canada)

Fax number: 314-447-8029

Elsevier Health Sciences Division
Subscription Customer Service
3251 Riverport Lane
Maryland Heights, MO 63043

*To ensure uninterrupted delivery of your subscription, please notify us at least 4 weeks in advance of move.

Printed and bound by CPI Group (UK) Ltd, Croydon, CR0 4YY

08/05/2025

01864693-0004

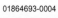